access

HEALTH *and* WELFARE

Janette Lloyd

Hodder & Stoughton

A MEMBER OF THE HODDER HEADLINE GROUP

Acknowledgements

With grateful thanks to the following for their help:

- Professor David Coggan of the Epidemiology Department, Southampton University Medical School for advice and for use of the hospital library
- Bob Digby for his initial help and Sue Warn for her constructive comments
- Mid-Hampshire Primary Care Trust for data
- Dr John Davies of St Clements Partnership, Winchester – my GP – for expert information and for keeping me in good health during this project
- My students on the Geography of Health course at Peter Symonds' College, Winchester for their enthusiastic suggestions
- Lastly, my twins, Jessica and Joseph, for their tolerance and support throughout

The front cover illustration is reproduced courtesy of S. Nagendra/Science Photo Library.

The publishers would like to thank the following individuals, institutions and companies for permission to reproduce copyright illustrations in this book: Punch, page 14; World Health Organisation, page 94.

Every effort has been made to trace and acknowledge ownership of copyright. The publishers will be glad to make suitable arrangements with any copyright holders whom it has not been possible to contact.

Orders: please contact Bookpoint Ltd, 130 Milton Park, Abingdon, Oxon OX14 4SB. Telephone: (44) 01235 827720. Fax: (44) 01235 400454. Lines are open from 9.00–6.00, Monday to Saturday, with a 24 hour message answering service. You can also order through our website www.hodderheadline.co.uk.

British Library Cataloguing in Publication Data
A catalogue record for this title is available from the British Library

ISBN 0 340 800291

First Published 2002
Impression Number   10 9 8 7 6 5 4 3 2 1
Year   2008 2007 2006 2005 2004 2003 2002

Typeset by Fakenham Photosetting Ltd, Fakenham, Norfolk.
Printed in Great Britain for Hodder & Stoughton Educational, a division of Hodder Headline Plc, 338 Euston Road, London NW1 3BH by Bath Press Ltd, Bath.

Contents

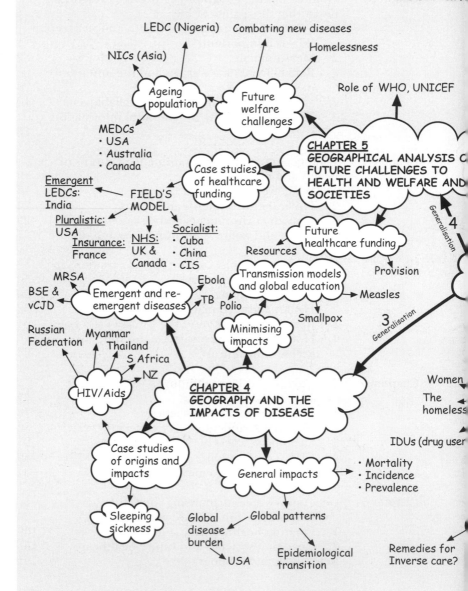

LEDC (Nigeria)   Combating new diseases

NICs (Asia)   Homelessness

Ageing population

Future welfare challenges

Role of WHO, UNICEF

MEDCs
• USA
• Australia
• Canada

Case studies of healthcare funding

CHAPTER 5
GEOGRAPHICAL ANALYSIS O
FUTURE CHALLENGES TO
HEALTH AND WELFARE AND
SOCIETIES

Emergent
LEDCs:
India

FIELD'S
MODEL

Pluralistic:
USA
Insurance:
France

NHS:
UK &
Canada

Socialist:
• Cuba
• China
• CIS

Future healthcare funding

Resources

Provision

MRSA

BSE &
vCJD

Emergent and re-emergent diseases

Ebola

TB Polio

Transmission models and global education

Measles

Smallpox

Generalisation

4

Generalisation

3

Russian
Federation

Myanmar
Thailand
S Africa
NZ

Minimising impacts

HIV/Aids

Women

The homeless

CHAPTER 4
GEOGRAPHY AND THE
IMPACTS OF DISEASE

IDUs (drug user

Case studies of origins and impacts

General impacts

• Mortality
• Incidence
• Prevalence

Sleeping sickness

Global disease burden

Global patterns

USA

Epidemiological transition

Remedies for
Inverse care?

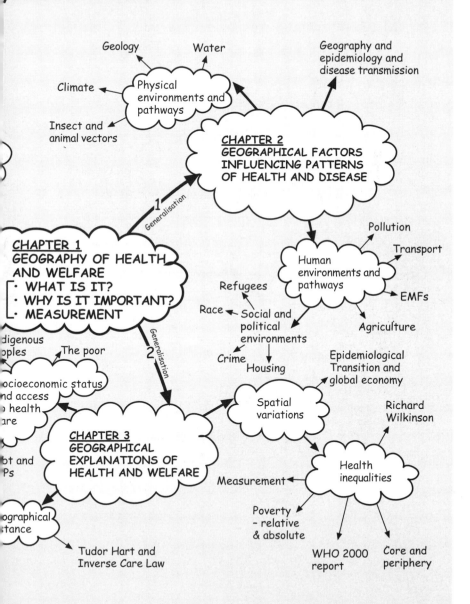

Geology   Water   Geography and epidemiology and disease transmission

Climate   Physical environments and pathways

Insect and animal vectors

CHAPTER 2 GEOGRAPHICAL FACTORS INFLUENCING PATTERNS OF HEALTH AND DISEASE

Generalisation 1

CHAPTER 1 GEOGRAPHY OF HEALTH AND WELFARE
- WHAT IS IT?
- WHY IS IT IMPORTANT?
- MEASUREMENT

Pollution   Transport

Human environments and pathways

Refugees   EMFs

Race ← Social and political environments   Agriculture

digenous ples   The poor

Crime   Housing   Epidemiological Transition and global economy

ocioeconomic status nd access health are

Generalisation 2

Spatial variations   Richard Wilkinson

CHAPTER 3 GEOGRAPHICAL EXPLANATIONS OF HEALTH AND WELFARE

bt and Ps

Measurement ← Health inequalities

ographical tance

Tudor Hart and Inverse Care Law

Poverty – relative & absolute

WHO 2000 report   Core and periphery

Researching Global Futures

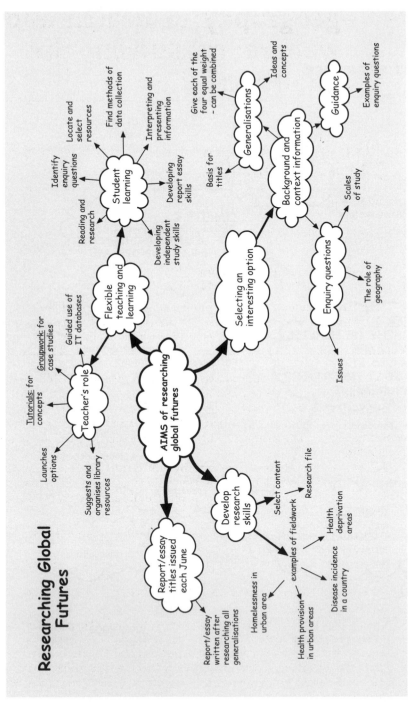

1 Foundation: the geography of health and welfare; measuring the quality of life

1 What is the geography of health and welfare? Why is it important?

> We're all of us ill in one way or another;
> We call it health when we find no symptom
> Of illness. Health is a relative term.
>
> > T.S. Eliot
>
> Life is not living, but living in health.
> > Martial – Roman poet 1st century AD
>
> Health is a state of complete physical, mental and social well-being and not merely the absence of diseases and infirmity.
> > World Health Organisation (WHO) charter 1946

Of the definitions of health above, the one from the WHO is most influential today, but all of them are important!

Geography is concerned with the interaction between humans and their environment. The issues which arise can be analysed over time (**chronologically**) and, more particularly, over an area (**spatially**).

The relationship between geography and health has been investigated for more than 50 years. Geographers are uniquely placed to analyse these issues since their subject embraces so many other disciplines:

- The geography of health investigates topics such as the pattern and spread of disease.
- Physical and human factors can greatly influence the health of the local population.
- Disease and infection have profound social economic and environmental effects.
- The quality of life varies greatly; welfare (a state of well-being) can be measured using a variety of indicators and scales.
- Poverty has a profound impact on all aspects of health and welfare.
- Each society responds differently to the challenge of providing healthcare and welfare for its members. The most expensive provision is not necessarily the best.

- The twenty-first century will present new challenges in the form of the emergence of virulent new diseases and a rapidly ageing population.

Through the study of all these topics, health geographers can make an important contribution to future plans and policies. This includes:

- advising on planning for healthcare staffing in those Southern African countries devastated by the HIV/AIDS crisis (as is being done by geographers from Southampton University);
- investigating the optimum pattern of healthcare provision in new Primary Health Trusts (in Mid-Hampshire for instance);
- analysing the global correlation between income and welfare;
- monitoring the effects of climatic change on the emergence of new infectious diseases;
- mapping the incidence of certain cancers to identify possible links between them and, for example, electro-magnetic fields or the occurrence of radon gas from igneous rocks.

2 Measurement

a) How helpful are traditional indicators of health status – morbidity (illness) and mortality (death)?

Basic data on the health of individuals and of populations (demographic data) is concerned with **morbidity** (illness) and with **mortality** (death) (Meade & Earickson 2000). It is normally expressed in rates (the frequency of one thing in relation to another over a particular period). It is best to use a specific section of the population if possible, as this gives a more accurate picture. When the total population is used, the rate is called the crude rate.

For example:

$$\text{Rate} = \frac{\text{Number of events in a given population for the specified time and place}}{\text{Total population at risk during the specified time in the specified place}}$$

The crude rate for mortality is:

$$\text{Crude mortality (death) rate} = \frac{\text{Number of deaths during year}}{\text{Total mid-year population}} \times K$$

The age specific mortality rate for those over 65 is:

$$\text{Over 65 mortality rate} =$$
$$\frac{\text{Number of deaths in population over 65 during year}}{\text{Mid-year number of those over 65}} \times K$$

K is a constant (usually 100, 1,000 or 100,000) used to turn the rates into whole numbers (per 1,000 for instance).

Other important rates are:

1. **Infant Mortality Rate (IMR):** the number of deaths occurring in children under one year. This is useful as it is a barometer of social and environmental conditions and is very sensitive to changes in either.

2. **Case Mortality Rate:** the number of people dying from a disease divided by the number of those diagnosed as having the disease.
3. **Attack Rate:** the number of cases diagnosed in an area, divided by the total mid-period population, over the period of an epidemic.

The use of **age–sex pyramids** to show the pattern of deaths is discussed by Cliff and Haggett (1988). Age–sex pyramids usually show the percentage of different age groups in the living population; using them to show mortality patterns is a novel approach. Since the population records in Iceland are very accurate, age–sex pyramids were used to investigate the effects of different groups of diseases. The resulting diagrams (Figure 1.1) illustrate:

- A – the standard population pyramid
- B – the age–sex pattern of all deaths showing that men tend to die at a younger age
- C and D – the age–sex pattern of deaths from cancer (neoplasms) and heart disease; D illustrates the tendency for men to contract heart disease at a younger age than women
- E – shows that 50% of deaths from this cause were the elderly dying from pneumonia in the winter months; the solid line shows that young children were also at risk
- F – shows the tendency for young males to die in road traffic accidents.

Apart from the IMR, these rates alone can give only a limited picture of the health status of an area. More specific data concerning lifestyle and living conditions are needed.

b) Do indicators of lifestyle and living conditions give a fuller picture?

The UK 2001 Census form contains the type of information on lifestyle and living conditions necessary for future health and welfare planning, in addition to giving an accurate idea of the state of the nation's health in April 2001. There are detailed sections related to:

1. **Household accommodation** – the number of rooms, including the number of baths and toilets and the availability of central heating.
2. **Family relationships** – showing single parent families and unmarried partners.
3. **Education** – especially important for the mother in the family as it influences her role as nurturer of the children.
4. **Self-estimate of health status and carer roles** – gives an idea of how well the respondents feel and whether they have a limiting long-term illness (including degenerative problems associated with ageing). It also identifies those who care for friends or relatives voluntarily. This is an important component of the informal welfare system, which was impossible to quantify hitherto.
5. **Employment details** – put into a new definition of social class,

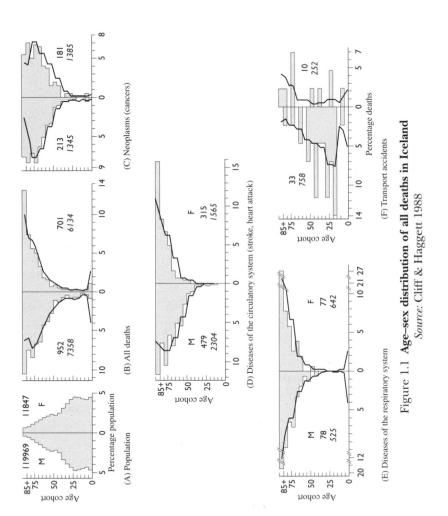

Figure 1.1 **Age–sex distribution of all deaths in Iceland**
Source: Cliff & Haggett 1988

enabling the correlations between working conditions and responsibility, for instance, and health status to be investigated. It is known that work-related stress occurs when there is little individual freedom in the workplace. Income levels have a strong influence on life expectancy.

6. **Car and house ownership** – can hint at the income levels of the household and indicate the need for planning public transport and housing strategies and possible pollution hazards.

Other **quantitative** lifestyle indicators such as calorie intake, consumer durable and telephone ownership can give a broader idea of the influences of lifestyle on an MEDC population's health status.

In LEDCs, literacy levels and school enrolments can also assist analysis.

On a broader scale, economic indicators such as **GNP per capita** (gross national product per head) and **GDP per capita** (gross domestic product per head) show the total value of goods and services produced by a country. This does not, of course, show how that income is distributed, which makes the study of the relationship with health indicators unrealistic on their own.

Another way of investigating living conditions is to use the **qualitative** approach. This measures characteristics, not actual quantities. **Environmental quality** (EQ) assesses the different components of the final score (access, vegetation and open space, building quality, for example) as penalty points. This data, usually derived from urban areas, can be the basis for **isoline mapping**. Point data concerning health from other sources could be used as a comparison. Hence low birthweight babies born in different sectors of a city could be related to EQ.

The levels of **crime** in a particular area also have an important effect on the social and, in some cases, the actual physical well-being of its inhabitants. Mapping 'the geography of fear' has been done for urban areas such as Manhattan Island in New York City. The lack of **social cohesion** in such areas is an important component in the pattern of **deprivation** and ultimately, **poor health**. Mapping those features of the **built environment** which encourage **crime potential**, such as unlit walkways and unattended lifts, was pioneered by Alice Coleman.

The use of all these indicators can be very helpful as general background, but by themselves they can give a simplified picture only.

c) Are service delivery (welfare) indicators a useful concept?

Again, these indicators can give a general picture of the availability of services which promote the general health and welfare of a population, but it is most important to realise that they are often equalised across a country or region. They do not take account of possible clustering in some places nor of uneven distribution (perhaps according to income levels) within the population. In addition, the definition of a particular service in the UK for example, such as the concept of a 'doctor' or a 'hospital' could well differ from its counterpart in the Russian Federation or in Sierra Leone.

Measures might include:

1. **General:**
   - Number of people per doctor
2. **Primary healthcare:**
   - GP consultations
3. **Secondary healthcare:**
   - Number of hospital beds per head of population
   - Hospital admissions
   - Hospital hygiene league tables
   - Waiting lists to see a consultant
4. **Welfare:**
   - Income support claimants
   - Unemployment claimants

In LEDCs this data would, of course, be scanty and unreliable at best.

d) Why are composite indicators necessary for analysis?

From all of the above it is clear that **single measures of health and welfare** are inadequate for any type of analysis in depth. The influences on health are so complex that it seems sensible to attempt to put some of the most important measures together as **composite indicators** in order to create a more accurate picture. The combination of social and economic variables can vary according to the area of study (in both senses of the word).

Carstairs (2000) discusses the use of the **deprivation index** (plural: indices), a composite indicator for the degree of poverty or affluence in the UK. Most of the material necessary is available from census data.

The deprivation index is derived from the view that being unemployed and living in crowded accommodation is worse than being employed and living in a spacious house with modern amenities (Gordon, quoted in Carstairs 2000). Characteristics such as wealth, higher social class and education are seen as the means of progressing from deprivation to affluence. There is a difference between **deprivation** (meaning the conditions suffered by people who are poor) and **poverty** (the lack of income preventing individuals from escaping from deprivation). As information about income is not available from the census, car and home ownership are included in indices as a measure of wealth. Car ownership is becoming more universal, and is essential in rural areas, so this is less useful as time progresses.

The following indices are commonly used by geographers, health statisticians and **epidemiologists** (scientists studying factors affecting the pattern and spread of disease):

1. **The Jarman index**, or underprivileged area (UPA) score, was derived specifically to assess the need for GP services (primary health care) but has more general use. The map of the Mid-Hampshire Primary Care Trust (Figure 5.7) shows how it can be used. It has been found to have a reasonably high correlation (0.70) with mortality and morbidity measures.

There is a wide range of individual indicators used in the main deprivation indices for health analysis (see Figure 1.2):

2. **The Carstairs index** The correlation with morbidity and mortality data is an impressively high 0.85.
3. **The Townsend index** The correlation with morbidity and mortality data was not as strong (0.70) as the Carstairs index.
4. **The Department of Trade, Environment and the Regions (DETR) index** The correlation with morbidity and mortality is 0.76.

When using deprivation scores it is usual to group the scores into

	CAR	JAR	TOWN	DETR
Unemployment (M + F)		3.34	X	X
male	X			
No car	X	X	X	
Low social class (IV/V)	X			
Unskilled (SEG11)		3.74		
Overcrowding	X	2.88	X	X
Not owner-occupied			X	
Lacking amenities				X
Single parent household		3.01		
Under age 5 years		4.64		
Pensioner living alone		6.62		
Moved in past year		2.68		
Ethnic minorities		2.50		
Children in unsuitable accommodation				X
Children in low earner households				X
Age 17 / not in education				X
Non-census variables				
SMR <75				X
Unemployed more than 1 year				X
Income support recipients				X
Low education level (GCSE D or less)				X
Derelict land				X

CAR, Carstairs; JAR, Jarman; TOWN, Townsend; DoE, Department of the Environment (now DETR) 1991.

Figure 1.2: **Main deprivation indices for health analysis**
(Source: Carstairs, V. Socioeconomic factors at area 1 level and their relationships with health in *Spatial Epidemiology*, Elliot, P., Wakefield, J., Best, N., & Briggs, D. O.U.P. 2000)

classes so that comparisons can be made. Some of the health variables related to deprivation have been found to be:

Mortality, Morbidity, Health behaviour, and Service use

These have all been investigated by the Trent Area Health Authority using the Townsend index (see Chapter 3).

On an international scale, **composite social indicators** such as:

1. the PQLI (Physical Quality of life Index), which combines life expectancy, infant mortality and adult literacy
2. the HDI (Human Development Index), using real income per capita, adult literacy and life expectancy at birth

can also be set against health variables. The drawback is the low economic input.

When using any of these measures it is important to bear in mind the following comments by Carstairs (2000):

Socio-economic position does not, of itself, explain health state; rather it represents a complex of living experience, living and working conditions, attitudes and social orientation, income wealth and assets for the individual ...'poor places' provide socially adverse environments that strike at the health status of even the non-poor inhabitants – many residents suffer from a combination of poor opportunities, poor services, sometimes high crime, low morale and stigma which compounds the individual experience of poverty.

In November 1998, the UK government introduced the so-called 'skylark index', which was part of a document called 'Sustainability Counts'. This attempted to establish indicators of **sustainable development** including indicators for:

- Economic growth – total output of the economy plus investment in public services and levels of employment
- Social progress – life expectancy, education and housing quality
- Environmental protection – climatic change, air pollution, road traffic, river water quality, housing on brownfield sites, and wild bird populations (hence 'skylark')
- Waste disposal.

The aims of the project were to:

1. make the indicators meaningful
2. relate them closely to sustainability targets for the UK.

Despite the criticism levelled at the project, the findings provide a good picture of quality of life for the UK. The 'best' area was judged to be North Yorkshire and the 'worst' was Knowsley on Merseyside. Thus, deprivation indices can be appreciated in a more general setting.

3 Reliability of data sources and the importance of scale

In London in 1632, John Graunt used tombstones and bills (records) of mortality to analyse causes of death (Meade & Earickson 2000). Although some of the diseases he mentioned, such as dropsie, jawfain and bloody flux, are obscure, of approximately 10,000 deaths, 1,800 were from consumption (TB) and 531 from smallpox.

Even in MEDCs today there might be some variation in the way that the causes of **mortality** are recorded. But the World Health Organisation issued a classification of diseases in 1993 which made standardisation easier. Even so, it has been estimated that the cause of death is sometimes misdiagnosed in up to 30 per cent of cases in MEDCs.

Morbidity (disease data) is less reliable. In the USA there are detailed sample surveys of morbidity. In the UK the new 2001 census gives some self-reporting on health status. Some diseases are so infectious that by law they must be reported; these are usually included in international surveillance programmes (see later in this chapter for details). Plague, cholera and yellow fever are the most serious, but malaria, influenza and typhoid are some other examples.

Where can I find relevant and reliable data?

Sources of data are increasingly easy to access from the appropriate web sites. As Meade & Earickson (2000) comment:

> Maps that could not be made from data that could not be analysed a decade ago are now free to download and print out in colour.

A bibliography and recommended references to websites will be found at the end of the book; here is a brief introduction:

1. Global scale data can be obtained from:
   - The World Health Organisation, which has a vast store of information for individual countries, too
   - The United Nations and UNICEF for population information
   - The World Bank – ECuity (European Union) and HNP (Health Nutrition and Population) projects
   - The US census bureau's international data base

2. Regional and national scale data from:
   - Demographic and Health surveys – provides a vast amount of demographic and health-related data for many countries
   - US census material
   - UK census and national statistics
   - UK HMSO – *Regional Trends* and *Social Trends*

3. Local data sources for the UK, for example:
    *   Primary care trusts (e.g. Mid-Hampshire, UK)
    *   Area Health Authorities (e.g. Trent or East London and the City, UK)

4. Journals, for example
    *   *New Scientist*
    *   *Geography Review*
    *   *Journal of Epidemiology and Community Health*

All the above are reliable sources of data, which can be analysed in a wide variety of ways to enhance case study material.

4 The part played by geographical information systems (GIS)

a) What is GIS?

GIS is a new and revolutionary way in which data can be collected, stored, manipulated and mapped. It allows complex interrelationships, which would have been impossible to create and to analyse until recently, to be built up gradually and accurately until the full picture is obtained. It can be used in:

*   computer cartography (mapping) with many different variables contributing to the final pattern
*   remote sensing from satellite photographs to provide accurate images of, for example, deforestation or water pollution
*   urban planning to analyse networks of roads or sewers, for instance.

Data goes into the system as co-ordinates or in a series of cells.

b) How does it work?

An example quoted in Meade & Earickson (2000) is that of the risk of environmental lead poisoning in a part of North Carolina, investigated by Hanchette in 1996.

*   Indicators associated with high lead risk were used instead.
*   They were: houses over 50 years old, population receiving public assistance, low house values, low incomes, single female parents, black population, rented housing and children in poverty.
*   Each of these was mapped as a choropleth map.
*   The final composite map represented high-risk areas for lead poisoning.
*   The addresses of children who had been found to have high blood levels of lead were superimposed upon the map.
*   Statistical analysis was done to see how well the map had predicted the pattern of lead poisoning.

Although it is clearly a powerful technique, it is most important to remember that the intelligent approach to GIS is that there is human input at all stages. This is valuable when deciding the nature of data required in the first place, but also in the type of map at the end. Meade & Earickson (2000) sum up

> And yet, the euphoria is real. Health researchers need to proceed with due care ...but the potentials are revolutionary.

Summary

1. 'Health is a state of complete physical, mental and social well-being and not merely the absence of disease and infirmity.' World Health Organisation charter 1946.
2. Geography is uniquely placed to analyse health issues. It is concerned with the interactions between humans and their environment, which are major determinants of health status. It can make an important contribution to future plans and policies for health and welfare services.
3. Traditional indicators of health are morbidity (illness) and mortality (death) rates. These and infant mortality and disease incidence rates are usually expressed in rates per 1,000.
4. Detailed quantitative information concerning lifestyle and living conditions in the UK can be obtained from the 2001 census. Data from LEDCs is less reliable. GNP and GDP figures are available worldwide but are of limited value in showing income distribution.
5. Qualitative data (related to characteristics rather than actual quantities) can be in the form of environmental quality, the geography of fear or crime potential.
6. Service delivery data such as the number of health personnel or facilities is of limited use in analysis if it does not have a spatial distribution.
7. Composite indicators attempt to analyse complex issues by putting several quantities together. A deprivation index attempts to quantify the conditions suffered by people who live in poverty. Such indices were developed in the UK. The UK 'skylark' index includes life expectancy in a composite indicator of regional sustainable development.
8. There are four main deprivation indices: Jarman (specifically related to GP (primary health care) delivery), Carstairs, Townsend and the DETR (government) indices. Each uses a different combination of indicators. The Carstairs index has the highest correlation with health variables such as life expectancy, smoking rates or GP consultations.
9. Data can be obtained from global to local scales from a variety of sources. Recognised organisations such as the World Health Organisation and UNICEF have large websites containing detailed and highly relevant information at all scales. Local sources are obviously easier to find and are more reliable in MEDCs (Primary Care Trust and Health Authority data, for instance).

10. (GIS) Geographical Information Systems is a new and invaluable tool for mapping and interpreting the complex factors which influence disease incidence or resource distribution.

What geographical factors influence patterns of health and disease?

1 What are geographical factors?

a) Geography and epidemiology

Any investigation of patterns of health and disease brings geography close to **epidemiology**. This is the science of the distribution, occurrence and spread of disease. Hence geographers find that they have much in common with epidemiologists in looking at disease trends over time and space.

The classic study by Dr John Snow in 1854 traced the source of a London cholera outbreak to one particular polluted pump in Soho. Noticing that this was in a hot summer, when people tended to drink quantities of water without first boiling it to make tea, which was the usual practice, he turned his attention to the water supply. Mapping the victims' houses produced a clear distribution which pinpointed the pump (Figure 2.1). It was the first example of this type of analysis. It also confirmed the supposition that cholera was a water-borne

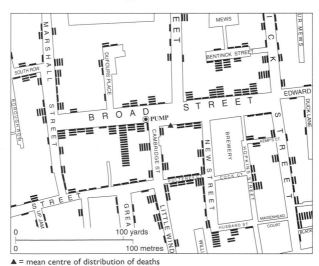

▲ = mean centre of distribution of deaths

Figure 2.1 **John Snow's map of deaths from cholera in Soho, London, 1854**
(redrawn)
(Source: Cliff, A. & Haggett, P., *Atlas of Disease Distributions*, Blackwell, Oxford 1988)

disease. A contemporary cartoon in *Punch* gives some idea of the quality London's water supply at the time (Figure 2.2).

The spread of diseases and their unequal global distribution can be related to a number of **geographical factors**, both physical and human. Jenkins (1999) suggests that population size, migration rates, transport routes and methods, in addition to the physical landscape, are all important. But the relationship between these is by no means straightforward. Influences that are not considered at first can turn out to be the most significant. Usually it is a complex interaction between many factors that underlies the pattern. This is particularly true of non-infectious and chronic diseases which, in turn, makes treatment and prevention much more difficult.

McMichael (1997) defines the environmental influences on health as:

the physical and chemical conditions in the living space around us, for example the quality of local urban air, fresh water supplies and the concentrations of chemical residues in food. A more liberal definition includes the conditions of the social environment – encompassing everything from housing quality

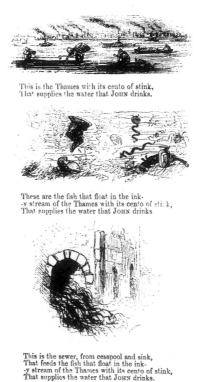

This is the Thames with its cento of stink,
That supplies the water that JOHN drinks.

These are the fish that float in the ink-
-y stream of the Thames with its cento of stink,
That supplies the water that JOHN drinks

This is the sewer, from cesspool and sink,
That feeds the fish that float in the ink-
-y stream of the Thames with its cento of stink,
That supplies the water that JOHN drinks.

Figure 2.2 **The water that John drinks**

to transport, recreational activities, population growth, density and mobility, social networks, and political and distributive equity.

b) Disease transmission theories

Infectious diseases have many causes:

- viruses such as 'flu or measles
- bacteria such as TB and meningitis
- fungus infections like athlete's foot and candida
- parasites such as tapeworms.

Insects and animals which carry the disease are known as vectors. Transmission occurs in a number of different ways, including:

- inhalation of droplets from coughs and sneezes, for example
- ingestion of contaminated food or water, for example
- skin penetration by mosquito bite or contaminated needle, for example.

The number of people affected by an infectious disease depends on two factors, according to Jenkins:

1. infection rate – the number of people infected by a disease in a given time
2. recovery rate – the number of people recovering from the infection over that time.

When the infection rate is higher than the recovery rate there is a rapid rise in the number of people who are infected. Where the number of people with the disease is significantly measurable at a national or regional level it is an **epidemic**. If the disease exists on an international level then it has reached the **pandemic** stage. This happens particularly when:

1. The population is susceptible to the disease, as nobody has encountered it before, so there is no immunity.
2. The population has a high mixing rate, with high population density and good communication links.

Chronological models

Kilbourne suggests **influenza** spreads out globally in waves. A seasonal pattern shows a higher incidence in winter and a lower one in summer (Figure 2.3) The waves decrease in size as the population becomes immune to one strain of the virus. With fewer and fewer 'susceptibles' the strain dies out and the waves lessen in height. This is shown by the graph of influenza cases charted by a GP in Gloucestershire over many years (Figure 2.4). But the virus is able to change its antigens, which means that the body's defence mechanism does not recognise it. A new strain can therefore begin the process of infection all over again.

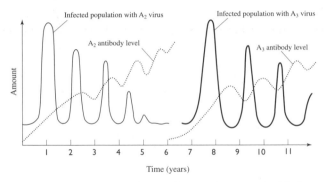

Figure 2.3 **Kilbourne's model applied to the spread of influenza**
(Source: Jenkins, S., 'Teaching about the geography of disease' in *Teaching Geography*, July 1999, Geographical Association)

This is the reason why it is difficult to immunise the vulnerable members of the population effectively. Complicating this picture is the fact that there are often several strains of influenza circulating at any one

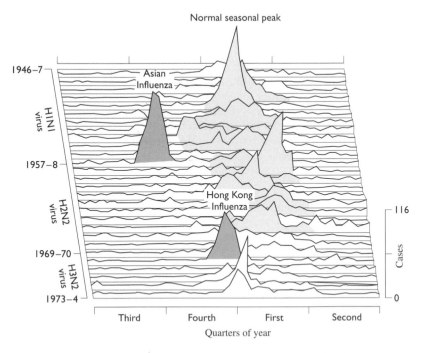

Figure 2.4 **The timing and intensity of influenza in Dr Hope-Simpson's Gloucestershire practice from 1946–7 to 1973–4**
(Source: Cliff, A. & Haggett, P. (op. cit.) 1988)

time. Sentiweb, a French website, produces animated maps of influenza patterns where the spread of the disease can be observed.

Jenkins describes Bartlett's model which examines the minimum number of people necessary in a population to support an **endemic disease** (one which is present at low levels in the population at all times). He found that a population above 250,000 could sustain endemic measles (Figure 2.5), by in-migration or birth of 'susceptibles'. Populations below this figure experience intermittent waves of measles as new infected subjects come into the area (ideally an island, where access is controlled), but very soon all are recovered and measles cannot be sustained unless re-introduced by outsiders.

Spatial models

The Hamer–Soper model looks at the spread of disease with the use of **demographic factors** of birth, death and in- and out-migration (Figure 2.6). Taking the example of an island, various situations are examined, involving **susceptible**, **infective** and **recovered** populations. Even at its most sophisticated, this over-simplifies reality. Mixing occurs irregularly and people vary in their susceptibility to disease.

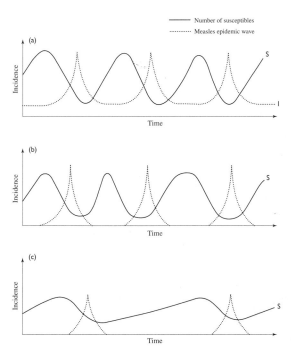

Figure 2.5 **Bartlett model a) stage 1 (population > 0.25 million) b) population < 0.25 million) and c) population very small**
(Source: Jenkins (op. cit.) 1999)

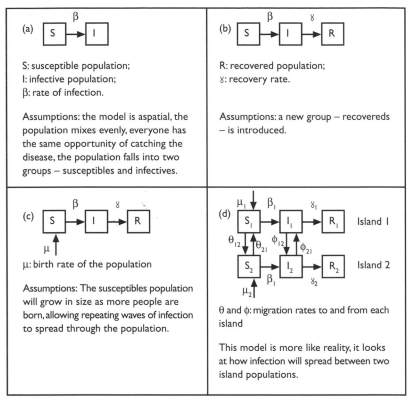

Figure 2.6 **The four Hamer–Sopel models a) model one – the most simple of the four – introduces the basic elements; b) model two – introduces factors which influence the spread; c) model three – introduces the idea that the susceptible population size will grow over time, and d) model four – more like reality, looks at how infection will spread between two island populations**
(Source: Jenkins (op. cit.) 1999)

Hagerstrand first identified **diffusion waves** when examining the spread of agricultural innovations amongst Swedish farmers in the 1950s (Figure 2.7). He stated that

- face-to-face contact was needed
- near neighbours were most influential in transmission
- new ideas were adopted as soon as they were heard about
- 'corridors' existed where spread was more rapid
- there were barriers to the spread (physical – for example, mountains and medical – for example, immunisation, in the disease model)

There are some ways in which these ideas do not transfer well to the epidemiological context. Diseases spread in a more complex manner

1) Expansion diffusion

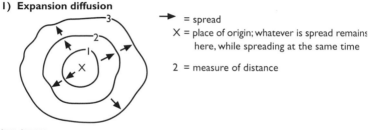

→ = spread
X = place of origin; whatever is spread remains here, while spreading at the same time

2 = measure of distance

two types:

a) contagious diffusion (spread by direct contact) – influenced by distance from place of origin. Risk lessens with distance.

b) hierarchic diffusion – spread through a class or group (e.g. different sizes of settlement)

2) Relocation diffusion

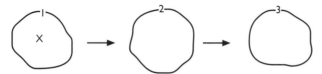

Whatever is diffusing shifts to a new place in time

3) Expansion/relocation combined

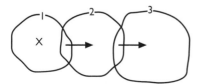

Both types occur simultaneously

Figure 2.7 **Types of diffusion**
(Source: Digby, B., *The Geography of Health*, Longman 16–19 Series, 1993)

than ideas. They do not always need face-to-face contact neither are always passed to neighbours.

Cliff and Haggett (Figure 2.8) describe the influence of **core-periphery** factors on disease transmission. The map shows the pattern of **influenza** in Northern England during one epidemic. The core obviously has urban areas with greater mixing rates. But on some occasions, it may be that the **focus** (source) of an epidemic is in a rural area and the infection travels from there to the core before being disseminated to rest of the periphery.

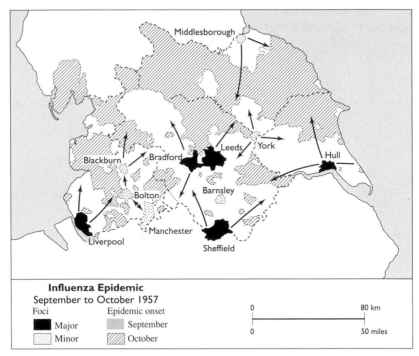

Figure 2.8 **Geographical path of the influenza pandemic of 1957 plotted for northern England**
(Source: Cliff, A. & Haggett, P. (op. cit.) 1988)

2 Physical environments and disease

The nature of the environment can be influential both for **infectious** and **non-infectious diseases**. In the former, it can provide ideal conditions for diseases to flourish. In the latter, it can be harmful or be deficient in the elements needed for healthy living. It can form a barrier to the spread of infection in the form of mountains or islands, or encourage it by flowing water. The geology and soil of a region, together with its climate and water supply, are fundamental factors in determining health status. Linked with this is the ecological setting, as this can provide a reservoir of **pathogens** and **vectors**. Humid tropical and equatorial environments can present the greatest risk and since many LEDCs are in this zone, the problems are often worsened.

a) Water

Access to clean water
Since the human body is to a large extent composed of water, it is essential to life. Water supply and water quality can thus be seen as

vital. The minimum human requirement to prevent dehydration is around 5 litres a day, but 30 litres is seen as the minimum for health, both for drinking water, cooking and for general cleanliness. In most MEDCs consumption per head is around 100–275 litres of clean water a day. About 40% of this is flushed down the lavatory. It is taken for granted that cheap and plentiful water is available for lawn-sprinklers, washing cars and swimming pools. There are regional shortages in some areas, especially those served by surface runoff rather than groundwater. Over 60% of the water supply for Los Angeles is imported from distances of up to 700 kilometres.

In Africa and central Asia particularly there are acute water short-ages, despite heavy rainfall and rivers prone to flood, so the access to safe drinking water is important. In many countries people (usually the women and girls) can spend hours collecting water, often carry-ing up to 25 litres on their heads for several kilometres, as in rural Zambia. In Jakarta, dwellers in kampongs (spontaneous settlements) might pay up to 40% of their income buying water from a private water-carrying service, as groundwater is too contaminated. Generally, public standpipes are cheaper than domestic supplies, but are less convenient. In Chennai (Madras) in India, about 2 million people use public standpipes, with each serving 240 people. In Dakar, Senegal, as many as 1,500 were using a single tap. Basic hygiene in these conditions is impossible, leading to the rapid spread of diseases, especially diarrhoea. Frequent illnesses of this kind enhance the vicious circle of poverty.

The lack of access to clean water is still widespread:

- in Africa, over 40% of the population is without clean water and over 50% without sanitation
- in Latin America the figures are 20% and 30%
- in Asia the figures are 30% and 40%.

Improving water supply and sanitation has been found to decrease IMR by an average of 55%. The problem for engineers seeking to improve the situation is, according to Cairncross (1997), that infections can be due to water-borne diseases or to poor hygiene due to lack of sufficient water. In Bangladesh, epidemiologists found that when they persuaded people to wash their hands to prevent faecal-oral disease transmission, dysentery incidence fell by 85%. People in Brazil who were instructed to chlorinate their stored water did not experience any drop in infec-tion rates as poor hygiene still prevailed. In-house connections are thought to be ideal, not least because they save many hours water carry-ing a day, as found by studies by the World Bank.

Water bodies
Both standing and running water, in tropical and equatorial areas particularly, present ideal opportunities for disease transmission, har-bouring vectors and parasites:

- standing pools of water can be habitats for the anopheles mosquito, the malaria vector and for the parasite drancunculus, which gives rise to Guinea worm
- irrigation canals contain the bilharzia (or schistosomiasis) parasite by snails
- running water can carry the larva of the black simulium fly, the vector for the parasitic worms causing onchocerciasis (river blindness), and the single-cell parasite giardiasis lamblia
- reservoirs, even in MEDCs , can be host to cryptosporidium, a single-cell parasite
- ponds and estuaries are the natural habitat of the cholera bacillus, vibrium cholerae, especially if they are alkaline and warm.

b) Geology

Radon
Radon gas is produced from the decay of uranium, naturally present in many types of rocks and environments. Igneous and metamorphic rocks and some mineral ores hold higher concentrations of the gas; their outcrops are areas of high exposure. The gas is colourless and odourless and can accumulate in buildings (which may also be constructed of the rock). Poor ventilation accentuates the concentration.

In Britain around 2,000 deaths a year from lung cancer are caused by radon. The National Radiological Protection Board's map identifies the areas of highest risk (generally levels of radioactivity exceed 100 bequerels per cubic metre). The gas can seep into wells. Tests in West Devon in 2000 found that 15% of all private water sources contained too much radon. Parts of Cornwall, Derbyshire and Northampton might also be affected. Radon in water is associated with an increased risk of stomach cancer, but it can be removed by an air-bubble filtering device.

In the United States, where nearly half the northern part of the country has an elevated risk of radon pollution, special radon-resistant building codes are in force.

In Romania radon from uranium mining was found to have significant effects on the birth rate in the area, compared with a similar control group not exposed to radon from the mine. The rate fell from 45% in 1963 to 9% in 1979, which corresponded with a 15-year exposure to mining. The figure has not changed markedly since (Rambiou et al 2000).

Iodine
Iodine is an element essential to the functioning of the thyroid gland, regulating growth and development. Lack of iodine causes an enlarged thyroid gland (**goitre** or **hypothyroidism**) and leads to sluggishness, stunted growth and mental retardation. Pregnant women with this condition are likely to miscarry or to give birth to a child with co-ordination difficulties and a reduced life expectancy.

Food is a major source of iodine but, as Pennington (1995) has shown, some areas which are hilly or prone to floods have heavily leached soils from which the iodine has been flushed. If the country does not have access to iodine-rich seafood and is without supplementary iodine sources, populations can be at risk on a large scale. The Lao People's Republic is:

- land-locked
- subject to heavy monsoon rains
- mountainous
- lacking supplements to a poor subsistence diet of rice
- too poor to supply proper healthcare to all its population (over 4.3 million).

UNICEF surveys in the early 1990s discovered very high **iodine deficiency disease** (IDD) rates there; in some communities 92% of the people had goitre. Approximately 65% of schoolchildren showed IDD symptoms. Only 5% had a normal intake of iodine. WHO and UNICEF found that about a third of the world's population were at risk from IDD, with 655 million suffering from goitre. The effects on infants meant that whole communities can be denied normal intelligence levels. Consequently, a UNICEF campaign was launched to eliminate IDD.

By 2000, 70% of households in LEDCs had been given access to iodised table-salt, which is the cheapest and most effective remedy for IDD, at a cost of around $69,000 million. More than 85 million newborn babies have been saved in this way, but in 30% of the targeted 82 developing countries still less than half the population use iodised salt. UNICEF had set the goal of eliminating IDD by 2000. Although this has not yet been reached, significant progress has been made.

c) Ozone depletion

Ozone deficiency in the stratosphere as a result of the use of CFC propellants in aerosol sprays has been well documented since the late 1970s. The UV-B (ultra-violet type B) surface radiation levels have risen correspondingly as the protective effects of ozone have diminished. Although the 'hole' in the ozone layer was first noted over the Antarctic, levels have begun to fall over the northern hemisphere too. It is a seasonal pattern, being at its worst in late winter and early spring, and there is a positive correlation with latitude, as Figure 2.9 shows.

Effects on health are related to the damage to DNA inflicted by UV-B radiation. The incidence of **melanomas** (skin cancers) has risen dramatically in many countries. In Australia, fair-skinned Caucasian types are at greatest risk, especially if they expose themselves irregularly to high doses of UV-B, for example on a sailing or fishing holiday, rather than regularly working outside (Armstrong 1986). There is no doubt that over-exposure to the sun as a child can trigger malig-

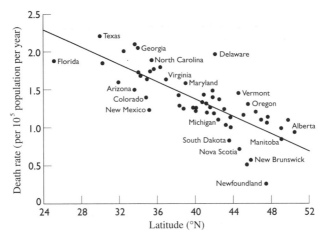

Figure 2.9 **The relationship of melanoma (skin cancer) to latitude in the USA and Canada**
(Source: Thomson, H. & Manuel, J., *Further Studies for Health*, Hodder, 1996)

nant changes in adult life. In addition, there is an increased risk of **cataracts** (thickening of the lens of the eye). Studies in Kuwait (Kollias et al 1986) showed that the darker pigments present in the indigenous population (by comparison with Europeans living in the country) were effective in reducing damage to the skin and eyes. The wearing of sunglasses without the correct lens filters is worse than wearing none, since the eye opens wider behind the dark lens, but is not protected from the increased ultra-violet light.

Paradoxically, Bentham (quoted by Henderson 2001) reported that people who live in sunny climates run a lower risk of developing multiple sclerosis, heart disease and strokes. This is due to the role of UV-B in producing vitamin D, which is beneficial in combating these conditions.

d) Ecology

We must extend our 'environmental health' definition to include the fundamental long-term role of ecological systems and processes as life-support systems. We are no longer talking only of an increased exposure to specific extraneous hazards as a cause of *bad* health. We are also recognising the depletion or disruption of natural biophysical processes that are the basic cause of sustaining *good* health. This includes...ecosystems...the hydrological cycle and the stratosphere 'ozone' shield against excessive solar radiation.

McMichael, T., 'Healthy world, healthy people', *People and the Planet*, 6:3, 1997

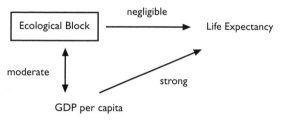

Figure 2.10 **Causal diagram describing the relationships among the E.I.
variables, GDP per capita and life expectancy**
(Source: *Epidemiology*, January 2001, Vol. 12 No. 1)

A possible relationship between the preservation of ecosystems and
health is shown on Figure 2.10. Sieswerda (2001) describes EI
(Ecological Integrity) as 'the ability of environmental life-support systems to sustain themselves in the face of human impacts'. The
relationship between EI and life expectancy was investigated for every
country in the world (203 countries), with the following variables
expressing EI:

1. percentage of disturbance by human activity
2. percentage of threatened species
3. percentage of protected species (to stand for biodiversity)
4. percentage of remaining forest (since agriculture began)
5. percentage of annual change in forest cover

The findings showed that the relationship between EI and life
expectancy was, in fact, controlled by many other (social, political and
economic) factors related to GDP. Many MEDCs can develop their
local resources far beyond carrying capacity by supplementing from
elsewhere. Warnings are given, however:

> there is a separation of consumption from consequence....At
> least in the short term, countries are rewarded for environmen-
> tal destruction with economic growth and ever-improving
> human health. If, however, the environment were unable to sus-
> tain an intense level of activity, human health would surely
> decline rapidly.

McMichael adds:

> As we acquire a more integrated view of the world's environ-
> ment, its ecosystems, and their fundamental role in sustaining
> the health of a growing population, so we must think more rad-
> ically about how best to manage and sustain these essential life-
> support systems.

e) Meteorology

Predicting the short-term direct and indirect effects of the weather on
mortality and morbidity rates is becoming more important in plan-

ning for health provision. A group of experts has been set up by the UK Meteorological Office to examine these impacts (Elkins 2000). By the analysis of a decade of data relating to GP call-outs and hospital admissions, the relationship of illness and weather patterns is to be investigated. By comparison with the rest of Europe, winter-related illness is especially linked to mortality in the UK, because of inadequate heating and clothing.

Trends so far identified:

1. An increase of 30% in cardiac and stroke victims whenever there is a change in environmental temperature of over 5°C or more, as the body takes between five and six hours to acclimatise; the blood thickens putting more strain on the heart and raising the blood pressure.
2. A similar increase in infections with a drop in temperature owing to the shock of the change. Chest infections from the air-borne RSV (Respiratory Syncytial Virus) peak just before Christmas, and seem to be associated with damp and foggy weather.
3. Low cloud and still air from an anticyclonic 'gloom' produces more influenza cases. The UK epidemic of 1989 occurred after four such days.
4. Thunderstorms precipitate asthma attacks; rates can increase by a factor of six.

Checkley et al (2000) examined the effects of the El Niño Southern Oscillation (ENSO) event and the associated temperature rise on the incidence of childhood **diarrhoea** in Lima, Peru. Admissions for Oral Rehydration Therapy (ORT) from 1993 to 1998 were used to analyse this relationship; a 200% rise was detected during the 5°C temperature increase in 1997–8. For each rise of one degree centigrade, the number of admissions increased by 8%; this was greatest during the winter. The epidemiological implications are that the increased frequency of this event will give rise to a large outbreaks of diarrhoeal diseases in similar areas.

f) Climatic change

Most researchers agree that the mean global temperature is due to rise by 6°C by 2100. This **global warming** will result in the polewards shift of the main climatic zones. The mid-latitudes will be stormier with hotter summers; lower latitudes could experience lower rainfall as desert margins spread further north and south. As the extent and timing of some of the changes will be on a very large scale (Haines et al 1993), impacts may be indirect and delayed.

Direct effects on health will be:

- increased heat stress leading to higher mortality from cardiovascular diseases (heart attacks)
- food poisoning
- a rise in mortality rates from extreme climatic events such as storms.

Secondary effects will include:
- 'tropical' diseases becoming more common in higher latitudes as their vectors are more able to survive
- more cases of malnutrition in lower latitudes due to desertification and salinisation,

Tertiary effects will follow, for example:
- conflict over fresh water supplies
- social and economic impacts of environmental refugees.

Numbers of some of those newly at risk from disease as a result of these changes have been estimated by the United Nations Environment Programme (UNEP):
- 2,100 million from malaria
- 600 million from bilharzia
- 86 million from onchocerciasis (river blindness)
- 50 million from trypanosomiasis (sleeping sickness).

Careful monitoring of all types of environmental change will be essential. For health issues to be addressed, health indicators must be linked to the broader picture throughout. The Inter-governmental Panel on Climatic Change (IPCC) has instituted the Global Climate Observing System (GCOS) which involves the co-operation of 80 international organisations. The following features will be observed:

1. Mortality rates from high temperatures using a weather stress index (WSI) and asthma (peaking in late summer) collected on a weekly basis to relate to temperature fluctuations.
2. Data showing environmental ill-health (deaths of plants and animals), using indicator species which are particularly environmentally sensitive. These may also be vectors (see next section).
3. Remote sensing of changes in vegetation indices, which have been found to be related to animal and vector habitats.
4. Monitoring of marine algae for cholera bacillus (vibrium cholerae) together with fish and shellfish poisoning.
5. Precipitation and runoff patterns – studied for 91 countries by the Global Runoff Data centre and the Global Environmental Monitoring Centre (GEMS) – run by WHO/UNEP- charting pollution.
6. Data on food supply, food access and well-being, mainly from Africa, coupled with 'greenness' indices from remote sensing.
7. Ozone levels (gauged by trace chlorine gas levels) and reports of different types of melanomas and cataract incidence.
8. Rapidly-expanding or new infectious disease reports (see Chapter 5).

Health professionals agree that greenhouse reduction is increasingly essential, following the Rio and Kyoto summits.

Research on the long-term effects of ENSO (Sari et al) show that both drought (in normally humid areas like Indonesia) and flood (in

Latin America) will be more likely. The possible impacts of such events are detailed on Figure 2.11.

g) Insect and animal vectors

It is more than 120 years since **arthropods** (jointed animals with external skeletons) were found to carry diseases. Viruses, bacteria, protozoa and worms all need a blood-sucking host. Thus arthropods are their **vectors** (carriers). Such vector-borne diseases as malaria, dengue fever, plague, filariasis, louse-born typhus, trypanosomiasis and leishmaniasis are thought to have caused a higher mortality than all other causes combined, from the seventeenth to the early twentieth century (Gubler 1998).

In the last 30 years there has been a rapid resurgence in the type of disease described above (see Chapter 5).

Changes in the habitat of the disease-carrying insects, both natural and anthropogenic (human-induced), will alter the disease incidence pattern accordingly.

The **tsetse fly** carries **trypanosomiasis** (sleeping sickness – see Chapter 5), affecting both animals and humans, through much of Africa between 15° North and 20° South. The use of draft animals is impossible where trypanosomiasis is found. The native game is immune but cannot be domesticated. In the opinion of Rogers (2000), the incidence of this disease prevented the development of an efficient sedentary agriculture and later, urban civilisation and hence rapid economic development over this part of Africa. This, in turn, led to poor nutrition and a lack of enterprise possibilities which is still evident today.

The **anopheles mosquito** kills 1 million children in the African continent through its transmission of **malaria**. Malaria, too, greatly hindered colonial expansion; Africa was called 'the White Man's Grave' in the nineteenth century. Sickle cell anaemia, a disease specific to the local population, is probably an adapted gene which can prevent malaria.

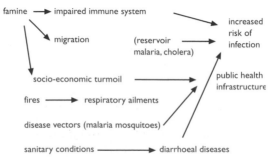

Figure 2.11 **Drought can affect human health via several pathways**
(Source: WHO : El Niño and Health 1999)

Many human diseases originally evolved from animals, with domestication. The species barrier was crossed as the diseases mutated. About 300 diseases had this beginning; 65 from dogs, 46 from sheep and goats and at least 35 from horses.

Wild animals also act as a reservoir for disease. The best-known example is the **black rat**, which has a tropical origin causing it to seek warmth and thereby closer association with humans when it migrates into temperate zones, usually aboard ships. Rat fleas transmitted the **bubonic plague** bacillus responsible for the Black Death in England in the late fourteenth century. Once it moved to humans it spread rapidly by droplets; domestic animals probably acted as reservoirs too. Wills (1996) suggests that the Great Plague in 1665 was less rampant in its effects because people lived more separately from their animals than did mediaeval peasants. Rats also carry rabies and typhus. Rat urine has been known to spread Weil's disease (leptosprirosis), in addition to Lassa Fever and Hantaviruses, both of which can be fatal.

Monkeys in sub-Saharan Africa have been associated with the deadly Marburg virus, otherwise known as Green Monkey disease, and could act as a reservoir for the Ebola virus, which often has fatal consequences (see Chapter 5). Bank voles in Russia are thought to harbour the kidney disease nephropathia epidemica.

3 Human environments and disease

There are many human modifications to the immediate living space and to the wider environment which have an effect on health. Those that are negative were not deliberate in the first instance, but since they are often indirectly related to health and are frequently associated with conflict or economic growth they can prove difficult to remedy. Small-scale impacts are worse in LEDCs or wherever the poor are victims, since they cannot afford to improve the situation by modifying their conditions or by migrating in search of something better. On a larger scale, the importance of international co-operation for positive change is vital, but this is often hard to achieve.

a) Transport routes

As people and goods move, so do the diseases which they carry with them. Vectors are mobile but do not move outside their habitats unless aided by different modes of transport. Tracing the mixing of populations that has occurred through each stage in transport innovation reveals greatly changing patterns of disease spread and distribution. The present speed and ease of travel means that the risks of infection have also increased. This is especially true of air travel which has enabled large volumes of movement worldwide.

Cliff and Haggett (1988) relate the spread of **cholera** directly to changes in international trade patterns. The focus (origin) of the

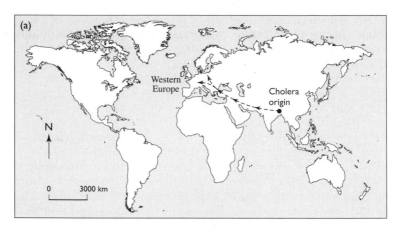

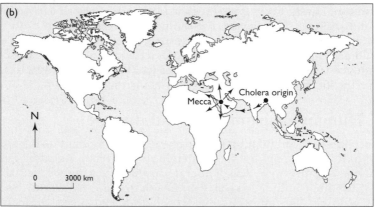

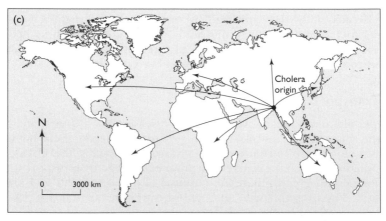

Figure 2.12 **The spread of cholera: a) phase 1 (first six pandemics), b) phase 2 (seventh pandemic) and phase 3 (eighth pandemic)**
(Source: Jenkins (op. cit.) 1999)

disease is in the Ganges delta area. It spreads fast because of its rapid incubation rate and because, being water-borne, it can contaminate the water supply of a whole area. Half the cases are dead within a week but treatment reduces the mortality rate to under 1%. Jusatz (1977) quotes evidence of eight global pandemics (Figure 2.12):

Phase one – the first six pandemics were confined to India until 1816. The disease then moved slowly across Asia with traders on foot, horseback or in sailing boats.

Phase two – the seventh cholera pandemic from 1965: cholera was mainly transmitted by sea. Pilgrims to and from the Muslim shrine at Mecca were the main carriers.

Phase three – the eighth pandemic, spread by air travel, was much more rapid.

The migration of millions of pilgrims to the holy festivals of Hinduism and Islam make a significant contribution to the spread of disease, but less so since vaccination has been introduced and great care is taken with sanitation and water supply arrangements.

The spread of **measles** was also greatly influenced by changing modes of transport. The virus has a 'life cycle' of 20 days. If the journey exceeds this time then all previously susceptible travellers will be in the recovery period when they arrive at their destination and thus not infectious.

The movement of the disease to the South Pacific is shown as a four-phase model by Cliff and Haggett (1988) (Figure 2.13):

Phase 1 – pre-virus contact: sailing ships from Europe took such a long time that the virus was dead before it reached the area.

Phase 2 – initial contact: steamships led to a shorter journey time; the virus survived, but the population was below 250,000; too low for it to become endemic.

Phase 3 – increased ease of travel: air travel increased, as did the population, so measles became endemic.

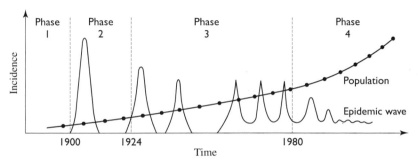

Figure 2.13 **Incidence of measles in the south-west Pacific**
(Source: Jenkins (op. cit.) 1999)

Phase 4 – vaccination: this programme meant that epidemics were less severe, although the disease remains endemic.

b) Pollution

All pollutants in the environment are potentially threatening to human health. Livermarsh (1993) lists the following types:

- chemical contaminants – from food contamination, pesticides, industrial accidents
- waste products – from hazardous waste, sewage, car fumes and indoor fumes from burning wood and dung
- non-ionising radiation (see next section).

In all cases, children are most at risk as they are growing rapidly and have a smaller body weight. Pregnant women can severely damage their unborn children by exposure to a variety of toxic substances. The elderly too, with less robust constitutions, are adversely affected.

McMichael (1997) quotes adverse health effects of extreme disasters such as those at Minamata (mercury poisoning of fish stocks in Japan), Bhopal (a chemical explosion which killed and blinded Indian villagers), Chernobyl (the explosion of a nuclear reactor in the Ukraine), and Love Canal (houses built on a toxic waste dump near Niagara Falls) as dramatic examples. But, more often, problems arise more gradually and may be difficult to trace as individuals can each experience different combinations of pollutants. This exposure might also be over a long period. Data collection and search for cause and effect is thus highly complex.

Some kinds of chemicals found in plastics, pesticides and industrial products, for instance, are weakly oestrogenic (Cadbury 1997), affecting female hormone balance. Others can modify androgens (male hormones) in addition to thyroid and adrenal gland function. The effects are worryingly widespread:

1. rising incidence of cancer of the testicles (300% increase in 50 years in Denmark)
2. rapid decline in human sperm counts (50% fall globally in 50 years)
3. dramatic rise in breast cancer (1 in 20 to 1 in 10 in the USA since 1950)
4. increase in prostate cancer.

But '…the significance of the findings for human health are still not known. For some, given the usefulness of the chemicals it would be irresponsible to ban them until we have further data. For others, given what we know now, it would be irresponsible not to ban them. This situation calls for an international treaty.'

Of all the types of pollution affecting human health, **air pollution** has the most widespread effects, as it can act on a variety of scales, from local to global. In addition it to being more mobile and potentially far more difficult to prevent and to control, there are many complex social and political factors involved. Globalisation means that transnational corporations can often operate with fewer restrictions on emissions and working conditions in poorer countries. This, in turn, has adverse effects on health, which may be immediate or delayed, and direct or indirect.

Most MEDCs now have many legislative controls in place, but it is the city dwellers in NICs and LEDCs who suffer most in the move to pursue economic development at all costs. Large numbers of poorly maintained vehicles, rapid industrial growth, few controls and the burning of open fires and inefficient stoves in spontaneous settlements combine to make filthy air.

In 1980, in Cubatao, Brazil, 40 out of every 1,000 babies were stillborn, and another 40 died within a week of birth, being mostly deformed (Philips 1993). In that year there were 10,000 medical emergencies involving TB, pneumonia, emphysema, asthma and other illnesses of the nose and throat. The total population was 80,000.

Also in Brazil, Gouveia (2000) studied the relationship between outdoor air pollution and mortality in São Paulo. All causes of death were investigated, and age and socio-economic status were taken into account. Most noticeable was the marked increased mortality in the elderly (over 65) associated with an increase in fine particulate matter (PM 10) and in sulphur dioxide. This was especially true of respiratory deaths. Cardiovascular deaths had a close association with carbon monoxide levels. In all cases it was the elderly in higher social groups who had the higher mortality rate. Gouveia suggests it was because they are 'protected' from other important causes of death by their status; air pollution is difficult to avoid. Curiously also, children seemed to be less vulnerable; possibly because they have been exposed to high pollution levels all their lives. Therefore, the severely polluted days had less impact on their health.

In most parts of the developing world, biomass fuels (wood, dung, grass and stubble) and coal are used daily for cooking and heating. As a result, indoor air pollution is often far worse than outdoor, especially for the women (Schwela 1997). The particulates, carbon monoxide, sulphur dioxide and nitrogen dioxide, released by combustion are carcinogenic and cause acute respiratory diseases. WHO estimates that 1.9 million deaths a year are due to indoor air pollution. The problem in tackling this issue is that it is part of traditional life and many cannot see it as a hazard and are not persuaded to install a basic, but efficient, stove instead.

Lanzhou, on the Yellow River in China (Hawkes et al 2001) was named as the world's most polluted place in 1998, since it lies in a mountain basin:

'Lanzhou is like a smoking room with no doors or windows,' said Yu Xionghou, director of the environmental protection bureau. 'There is no draught to clear out the smoke....if we weren't surrounded by smoke it wouldn't be any worse than any other Chinese cities.'

Lanzhou lies in a narrow valley ...which stretches for 25 miles and in places is as narrow a one and a half miles. Pollution from hundreds of chimneys and domestic fires produces a choking mixture ...the air is dusty and the elevation of the city makes the fumes from coal furnaces dissipate only slowly ...a radical solution is to demolish a 300m mountain to let in some fresh air ... but even a modest hill takes quite a lot of shifting. It is also trying some traditional methods; planting trees to absorb dust, converting coal-fired furnaces to gas and closing some of the dirtiest factories ...the city still has to endure 20 weeks of highly polluted air every year. Many people resort to wearing smog masks.

In Poland a study of pollution and health between 1985 and 1990 revealed 22 urban hazard areas, including Warsaw and Krakow. Due to factories like the Nova Huta steelworks near Krakow (which was built to an out-moded design, without emission controls, in the Soviet era) much of the country, especially Upper Silesia, was declared an ecological disaster zone. The air contained appallingly high lead and other particulate matter, and nitrogen dioxide concentrations were way above the internationally recommended amounts. The effects on the children meant that babies were born small for gestation dates, were often brain damaged and, if not, had a one in three chance of being chronically sick by the age of 10. Leukaemia cases were very much above the mean European figure. Since then, there has been stricter environmental control of air quality, and life expectancy has actually risen.

In Malaysia, a study was made comparing the frequency of asthma attacks in children in the polluted city of Kuala Lumpur with children in Terengganu, which is less polluted (Hashim 2000). Significant correlations were found between attack frequency and particulate matter, nitrogen dioxide levels, sulphur dioxide and ozone; these contributed to 71% of the attacks. The others were caused by different triggers.

Even in MEDCs there are still serious problems. Studies in Dusseldorf, Germany (Kramer 2000) identified nitrogen dioxide pollution as an extra trigger for atopic eczema incidence. Nyberg et al (2000) found that 20 years of exposure to nitrogen dioxide from traffic in Stockholm, Sweden, was a major cause of lung cancer. Ritz (2000) in California concluded that particulate matter and carbon monoxide concentration may contribute to the occurrence of premature births.

Studies in the Arctic (Lean 1997) have found high concentrations of polychlorbiphenyls (PCBs) and pesticides in the bodies of people living in very remote areas off Baffin Island. These are volatile enough to be carried from where they are used in the tropics (on rice paddies in India, for example) in the upper atmosphere until they condense over areas in high latitudes such as Greenland.

They concentrate in the Arctic because it is a relatively small area and the cold and winter dark slow down their natural degradation. And thus the peoples of the Arctic, who have contributed almost nothing to the pollution and do not benefit from the use of the chemicals thousands of miles away, become its principal victims.

c) Electro-magnetic fields

There are many types of **electro-magnetic radiation (EMR)**. Light is at one end of the spectrum, but **non-ionising radiation**, at the other end, is thought by some to be harmful to health (Powell 2001). Early research in the 1970s found that EMR above a certain strength could heat up human tissue. This could be associated with sleep disorders and threats to the immune system. Prolonged exposure could disturb calcium absorption and thus upset melatonin balance, which regulates the human 'body clock'.

There have been reports of large clusters of people living close to transmission masts developing **leukaemia** and other types of cancer. In 1999, an investigation by Professor Gordon Stewart at Glasgow University reported a 33% increase in cancer in people living close to television masts. Epidemiological studies by Henshaw (1998) appear to have established a statistical link between high electro-magnetic field (EMF) levels and childhood leukaemia. The causative mechanism rests on the ways in which EMFs influence carcinogenic aerosol pollutants:

- they cause them to adhere to the skin more readily
- they cause them to congregate
- charges coming from the power lines interact with the pollutants making them 'stickier', finer and more able to adhere to the lungs.

These effects have been found up to 5 kilometres from power lines. The UK Childhood Cancer Study (UKCCS) found increased childhood cancer in proximity to high-voltage power lines. The increased risks of the onset of Alzheimer's disease have also been noted.

Mobile phone masts are thought to have similar effects, which is a matter of grave concern for those communities, usually on hilly urban fringes, where phone companies wish to site them. Since the masts are often near schools and hospitals, fears are raised still further. A group of residents in Winchester, UK, (Winchester Extra February 2001) protested against an 11-metre mast which was to be erected at the end of their road adjacent to Western Primary School. There was no legislation to enable them to complain about the proposal, as the mast was under 15 metres high. Three other sites were proposed in the city but protestors favoured all the masts being on one site at some distance from buildings. The local MP was engaged in talks with the police authority about re-siting. The mobile phone company was also engaged in seeking planning permission for many new masts throughout the country, despite health fears.

d) Farming practices

Future Harvest, a non-governmental organisation (NGO) working for sustainable agriculture in the developing world states:

> more than 800 million people in the world go to bed hungry every night; they are chronically undernourished.... Every year nearly 13 million children die before the age of five as the result of hunger and malnutrition. In an ugly irony, as desperate farmers try to increase their production, their agricultural methods may contribute to more health problems. A farmer may overuse pesticides ...some methods of irrigation encourage the spread of human disease ...malaria and schistosomiasis ...

A particularly severe **famine** began to take hold in North Korea in the mid 1990s. This is very much a 'closed' communist society, unlike its NIC neighbour. By 2000, the situation was desperate for many people, even though reports were limited. Valfells (2000) visiting the worst-hit areas in the industrial north for the International Red Cross noted that people in the countryside were harvesting wild grasses for food. In the towns the situation was very bad:

> You don't have large-scale movements between different parts of the country. People tend to stay in their own ...province. We visited the town of Wee Chong, and there you have people starving silently on the seventh floor of apartment buildings. And they're starving because there is no food coming into the city ... there is no fuel left ...the coal mines were flooded ...industrial production is at a standstill ...there is no food coming from the countryside because it has been affected by natural disasters – floods and drought – and this means there is just enough to feed the people in the countryside, and even there you may see cases of malnutrition.

> It's especially the old people and the children who are affected ...the three year olds are smaller and not as developed mentally or physically as they should be at that age...it's affecting a whole generation.

By 2010 (Madeley 1995) predicts, despite expected food output increases in many of the LEDCs, '...the African continent may have 300 million undernourished people; 32% of its population...'.

Over-intensive agriculture in MEDCs has also produced health risks, for example the **salmonella** (a virus causing severe gastroenteritis) in eggs scare, the **e.coli** contamination of meat in slaughter houses in Scotland and, of course, the feeding of contaminated animal remains to other animals (naturally herbivorous, like cattle) which gave rise to the problem of **BSE** (see Chapter 4). Hormone growth promoters in beef cattle, which have been banned in the UK for 11 years, are known to contain carcinogens, in addition to rendering some men sub-fertile as the hormone finds its way into local groundwater and hence into the human food chain.

The other major concern is the effects of **Genetic Modification (GM)** (Soil Association 1999) of plants and animals on human health. Its supporters say that by selectively breeding a protection against a particular pest, the amount of toxic chemicals on the fields can be reduced. Its critics, especially Pusztai, quote the evidence of rats fed on GM potatoes. This revealed adverse effects on the rats' immune systems and damage to vital organs after only ten days. Some argue that Pusztai's results were flawed. Whatever the truth, there has been considerable opposition to field trials of GM cereals in the UK by one of the biggest GM companies. The irony is that there can be no real appraisal of the effects of the crops on the local ecosystems' gene pool without the trials. The Soil Association in the UK is campaigning for sustainable organic farming and is urging the World Trade Organisation (WTO) to consider a global ban on GM.

Three fundamental issues are important in future farming for famine avoidance (Hinrichsen 1998):

1. the need to slow population growth while promoting *sustainable* food production
2. increasing access to food supplies for the most vulnerable (women and children in LEDCs)
3. tackling absolute poverty (leading to poor diet and malnourishment) with sustainable agriculture and water use.

4 Social and political environments and disease

a) Refugees and civil war

Mass migration of people in civil wars is invariably linked to high morbidity and mortality rates.

Rwanda was plunged into war and genocide following the massacre of the Tutsi people by the Hutu people, and the reversal of the situation occurred when rebels overthrew the government in 1994 (Towfighi 1999). Around 800,000 died. Those Hutus who survived fled over the border to Zaire; a major camp was set up in Goma.

The crude mortality rate (CMR) in the camp was 30/10,000 *per day* compared with a pre-war figure of 0.6/10,000. Unaccompanied children were dying at a rate of 100/10,000 per day and babies at 600/10,000, mainly from diarrhoeal diseases, which made up 90% of the deaths.

The main reasons for this situation were:

1. lack of clean water – a polluted lake was the only source
2. poor sanitation – the ground was too rocky to dig deep holes for latrines
3. no adequate burial facilities – too rocky, so bodies were left by the roadside for transportation to mass graves.

The main health threats facing the refugees were:

- infection – especially air-borne diseases like measles, respiratory infections and meningitis, and those transmitted by faecal matter such as cholera, typhus and dysentery
- malnutrition – through lack of energy and protein; also scurvy, pellagra, beriberi and anaemia.

More than 45,000 died of cholera (from the lake) and 600,000 were infected within only three weeks. There was then a dysentery outbreak, and the children also contracted malaria and pneumonia.

Malnutrition was difficult to remedy, as the Tutsi political leaders in Rwanda blocked food supplies in retaliation for the earlier bloodshed.

Medical assistance followed the four levels of prevention set up by the International Red Cross:

1. Primary prevention – by vaccination, especially for children under five (for measles but not for cholera, since a clean water supply is more effective at first).
2. Secondary measures – sanitation and prevention measures such as distributing mosquito nets, education about basic hygiene, chlorination of water supplies and Oral Re-hydration Therapy (ORT).
3. Tertiary prevention – rehabilitation following illness such as high-energy diets after diarrhoeal illness.
4. Curative action – treating preventable diseases such as giving antibiotics for cholera to prevent it spreading.

By the third week a group of NGOs had moved into action. The UNHCR, NICEF and the Centre for Diarrhoeal Disease Control (Bangladesh) set up treatment centres. Their efforts significantly curbed the spread of disease. There were some problems in getting the operation working smoothly, which stemmed from there being too few workers at first. This meant that it was hard to give medical attention to all those who needed it. Some procedures, such as making up ORT solutions to the correct dilution, occurred. Finally, the relief workers had great difficulty obtaining enough pure water.

Lessons learnt from this tragedy can now be applied to all future refugee migrations:

- there must be enough relief workers available in place at the very start of a mass migration
- the workers must have a knowledge of basic management of diarrhoeal diseases

- special care must be taken to give help to those too sick to reach the medical posts
- appropriate antibiotics must be used
- chlorination of water must take place immediately a settlement is started.

Application of the above would have saved 50,000 lives.

b) Poor housing

Evans et al (2000) list those aspects of housing which have adverse effects on health:

- Generally, poor housing is linked health problems – and increased mortality.
- Nitrogen oxides from gas appliances can increase asthmatic symptoms; the carbon monoxide from a poorly functioning appliance can cause serious illness or death.
- Lead poisoning from old paintwork or plumbing can cause children to have lower IQ levels if exposed to lead. In adults, high blood levels of lead increase blood pressure.

A study by Lang (1997) of housing in seven US cities found the least adequate housing in inner cities and in the rented sector: 'Good housing is important for its beneficial impact on health and well-being.' New York had 12% of its housing stock judged as inadequate; St Louis, San Diego and Seattle had only 3%. New York had the highest rate of overcrowding – more than one person to a room (over 5%). This was more likely to be rented accommodation often inhabited by Hispanics or blacks. Of its inner-city housing, 14% was structurally inadequate compared with only 3% of suburban housing.

Blane et al (2000) have suggested that there is an 'inverse housing law' in the UK (see Chapter 3 for details of the *Inverse Care Law*). This links climate, housing and health by asking two questions:

1. Is there a mismatch between severity of climate and adequacy of construction methods so as to provide protection from cold and damp?
2. If there is a mismatch, is it associated with poor respiratory health?

Using GIS average rainfall and temperature for each county, a composite score was obtained to measure how warm and dry each was. The following data from the Health and Lifestyle Study was used similarly for a composite score:

- type of area
- housing tenure
- crowding
- outdoor or indoor toilet
- sole use of basic domestic facilities or not
- temperature in the living room
- indoor carbon monoxide levels.

Lung function was also tested and compared with the ideal readings for each person tested.

The main points to emerge were that:

- housing quality in Britain seems to vary inversely with the demands of the climate – that is, the harsher the climate, the worse the house;
- the greater the difference between the adequacy of the house, the worse the lung function;
- to target poor-quality houses in areas of harsh climate is the best way to tackle respiratory health and to narrow health inequalities.

The results are shown on Figure 2.14.

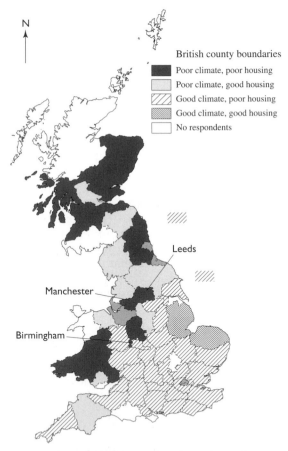

Figure 2.14 **Climate–housing mismatch**
(Source: Blane, Mitchell & Bartley 2000 Journal of Epidemiology and Community Health (www.jech.com))

c) Crime

The occurrence of crime, be it petty theft or more serious offences such as violence or even murder, can be linked to a number of geographical factors, including the **quality of life**. This, in turn, relates to **specific welfare indicators**, such as housing quality, unemployment rates and population structures. The resulting influences on the health of the local population can encompass mental health as well as the very real threat of physical injury.

The Washington DC Police Department mapped the density of homicide locations in the city in the mid-1990s in relation to population density, vacant housing and areas where the population lived below the poverty level. The resultant patterns clearly show that these phenomena co-incide, thus linking deprivation and poor environmental quality with violence in cities.

The Health of Londoners Project lists young offenders convicted in 1996. The location of burglary offences fits in with the general pattern of deprived inner boroughs and privileged outer ones:

- **inner boroughs** – for example, Greenwich, Lambeth, Newham and Tower Hamlets, have a mean figure of 250 young offenders accused of burglary
- **outer boroughs** – for example, Bromley, Harrow and Richmond, have a mean figure of 90 young offenders accused of burglary.

The second highest figure is from Southwark (252) which in turn is in the top third for violent young offenders (116 accused). The North Peckham Estate, which has figured greatly in the news as a dangerous place, is described variously as:

a desolate south London sink estate ...conditions within its slimy walls beggar belief ...in the eight weeks since contractors started demolishing the older part of the estate, they have found more than 20,000 hypodermic needles ...by the time it is dark the walkways are full of hooded youths screaming and fighting ...in two months there have been two murders and a kidnapping. Come nightfall, it is a complete no-go area'

Reid et al, *The Times*, 29 November 2000

the sprawling mass of condemned 1960s housing and gleaming low-rise blocks that are taking their place ...one of the most deprived estates in one of most deprived of inner city areas in Britain'

Sengupta et al, *The Independent*, 29 November 2000

The borough certainly has all the hallmarks of deprivation:

- 87% of the housing is rented from the local authority
- only one in four households has a car
- 30% of the population is under 16 years of age

- lone parents make up 16% of all households
- 57% of the population are from black and other ethnic minorities; Africans make up one quarter of this (the highest proportion of any community in the UK).

It is not surprising that there are particular health and welfare problems here, for example:

- the local health authority has experienced a rise of HIV cases to 10 times the national average
- 20% of all the sexually transmitted disease sufferers in London live in the borough
- the figures for teenage pregnancy are some of the highest in the UK
- many children are eligible for free school meals and the recent 'fruit supplement' pilot scheme
- the only remaining shop was due to close when demolition was completed. From 1993 until 2000 it was burgled 23 times.

By comparison, houses in the comparatively wealthy county of Hampshire and the Isle of Wight have half the mean risk of burglary for the UK in 2000 at an average of 20 a day for 740,00 households. This is 54% less than in 1992–3.

The national reduction in burglary statistics was 6% over this time. Those most at risk of crime, according to the Home Office report in 1999, are single parents living with children, young households (such as students) and those in inner cities (experiencing 10% of all crimes compared with 6% for rural dwellers).

The UK government has invested £50 million since 1997 on reducing burglaries (Research Development and Statistics Directive – Home Office 1999). The study found that there were certain characteristics which generated burglary:

1. **Related to the offenders** – a concentration of 'problem families' or cheap rented accommodation, for instance.
2. **Related to the victims** – a large number of naïve individuals with high-value items (students?) in an area.
3. **Related to the community** – low levels of informal control with high levels of unemployment and economic deprivation.
4. **Related to the type of buildings** – poorly designed estates with limited views and a network of alleyways (Radburn planning), terraced houses with back alleys, housing in multiple occupation, poor security locks and poor street lighting.
5. **Related to the location** – leisure facilities, for example football grounds or shopping facilities, drawing crowds of potential offenders with good transport links, or declining seaside towns with a large number of new migrants using illegal drugs.

Figure 2.15 gives two case histories of areas investigated by the study group.

CASE ONE: MIXING THE OLD AND THE NEW – VICTORIAN TERRACES OCCUPIED BY STUDENTS

The target area is adjacent to the town centre of a university town. The area is bisected by a major shopping street leading into the city centre, which evidently draws in large numbers at night-times. Here, the key generators of burglary are:

• a victim group (students) that is not particularly security conscious
• a good supply of attractive goods for theft (students' electrical goods)
• a supply of likely offenders living in the area
• housing design with limited capacity for surveillance at rear.

CASE TWO: THE TWILIGHT WORLD OF BED-SIT LAND

This area is in a striving holiday town with a population of 30,000. The town has clearly fallen on hard times, having lost its position as a popular resort, and found no significant replacement to holiday trade. Unemployment is high at around 20%.
In this area, the key generators of crime are considered to be:

• a transient population, living in relative anonymity, reducing the potential for effective natural surveillance
• a supply of HIMOs, that commonly consist of shared hallways and corridors where it is not unusual to see strangers
• housing provision that attracts socio-economic groups most at risk of engaging in burglary
• a local drug culture that may fuel property crime in the area.

Figure 2.15 **Case studies for burglary prevention**
(Source: Research Development and Statistics Directive Home Office 1999)

A survey carried out by the Dutch Ministry of Justice, quoted in *The Economist* in 2001, compared reports from those who were victims of different types of crime in seventeen countries. England and Wales were in the worst group with Australia, the Netherlands and Sweden. The countries most free of crime were Finland, Switzerland and Japan. The types of crime listed were:

• violent crime – the UK came second, behind Australia
• car theft – the UK was first
• burglary – the UK came second, after Australia.

Heavy drinking among young men is thought to be the reason for the violence. Houses in the UK have more burglar alarms than any

European country except Portugal. The reasons for the other results would seem to be increased social mobility and urbanisation.

d) Race

Ethnic groups are not only frequent sufferers when it comes to the allocation of health resources but they also have very different susceptibilities to a whole range of diseases.

Research carried out by Whitehead (1992) and Culley et al (1993) on ethnic groups in the UK found the following racial groups were particularly prone to a range of conditions:

Place of origin
- Africa – higher rates of strokes, high blood pressure, maternal deaths, TB, sickle cell anaemia
- Indian sub-continent (South Asian) – higher rates of diabetes, TB, liver cancer, maternal deaths, heart disease, thalassaemia
- Caribbean – higher rates of strokes, diabetes, sickle cell anaemia.

The South Asian population in the UK, for instance, does have other risk factors associated with its disease profile in addition to those in the UK population as a whole, according to research findings quoted in the British Heart Foundation (BHF) Bulletin 1997.

Part of the reason seems to be that the traditional labouring way of life in the Indian sub-continent, with a degree of under-nourishment, offsets the genetic pre-disposition. When people come to the UK, they adopt a more sedentary Western lifestyle in activity levels and diet, and the diabetes becomes a problem. The South Asian community in general takes little exercise, which makes matters worse. Compounding this is the change in diet, from a healthy South Asian diet to one with more sugar, fat and junk foods. With diabetes comes the risk of coronary heart disease, as it promotes high blood pressure and high cholesterol. Smoking makes the risks even greater.

Seeking medical attention can be a problem because of language and cultural values. The BHF has started a range of initiatives to tackle these problems, aided by the Department of Health. As part of the National Strategy for Neighbourhood Renewal, announced at the end of 2000, the government is pledged to aim for racial equality in service delivery for health and social services. It will tackle the problem of HIV/AIDS in black communities and attempt to appoint more ethnic minorities in the NHS.

The Healthy People 2000 initiative in the USA, begun in the early 1990s, aims to reduce health disparities between Americans. The differences in life expectancy, causes of death, numbers with health insurance cover and use of clinical preventive services are still marked, however, (1996 statistics) for example:

- The IMR for whites is 7.3/1,000 live births, for blacks 14.7/1,000, for Native Americans 10.0/1,000.

Stroke deaths, 1996

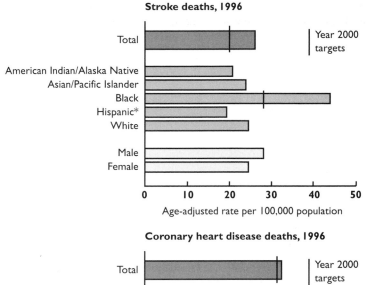

Age-adjusted rate per 100,000 population

Coronary heart disease deaths, 1996

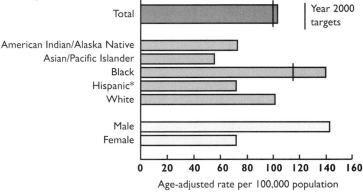

Age-adjusted rate per 100,000 population

Death rates are age-adjusted to the 1940 US standard population.
* = Persons of Hispanic origin may be of any race.

Figure 2.16 **US stroke deaths and coronary heart disease deaths 1996 and**
2000 totals
(Source: US CDC department 2000 www.cdc.gov)

- Cardiovascular deaths were 163.6/100,000 population for whites, for blacks 251.0/100,000, for Native Americans 128.1/100,000.
- Incidence of AIDS for whites was 13.4/100,000, for blacks 110.9/100,000, for Native Americans 13.4/100,000.

Objectives for strokes and coronary heart disease, which were set for 2000, are shown in Figure 2.16. The project is still running, with the next objectives set for 2010.

Summary

1. Epidemiology is the science of the spread and pattern of disease, and is therefore closely linked to geography. A number of physical and human factors influence this spread and pattern, including geology, climate, ecology, population size, migration, transport routes, conflict, environmental quality, and race. Their interaction can be complex.
2. Theories of infectious disease transmission can help the understanding of epidemics and pandemics (measures of the incidence of diseases in populations). They are mainly chronological – for example, 'waves' of influenza over the winter, or mainly spatial – for example, the diffusion of a disease throughout an area.
3. Many people in the developing world lack access to clean water, which means that they are especially prone to diarrhoeal diseases. Water can also act as the breeding ground for parasites and vectors (carriers) of disease, particularly in tropical environments.
4. Radon gas, produced by the decay of radioactive minerals in igneous rocks, can give rise to cancer. Lack of iodine in heavily leached soils in mountainous areas without access to the sea means the risk of iodine deficiency disease. This causes low intelligence and tiredness. Miscarriages and foetal abnormalities are also a result.
5. The 'hole' in the ozone layer makes skin cancer more likely in high latitudes and among fair-skinned people. It is possible to relate illnesses such as strokes, influenza, chest infections, asthma and diarrhoea to short-term variations in temperature.
6. Climatic change associated with global warming will bring a number of effects, such as the poleward migration of tropical diseases.
7. Ecological damage will eventually have adverse influences on human populations.
8. Many tropical infections (viruses, bacteria, protozoa and worms) are carried by vectors, usually blood-sucking insects. Their distribution governs the pattern of the diseases that they carry. Animals such as the rat and the monkey can be reservoirs of disease by acting as hosts to vectors.
9. Transport routes and the mode of transport have a direct relationship with the rate and pattern of the spread of disease. Cholera pandemics can be related to changes in transport modes. Measles has reached new parts of the world as transport has become more rapid.
10. Pollution from chemicals in pesticides and fuels, for instance, has had a devastating effect on human health. Cancer and infertility are two known problems.
11. Air pollution is particularly devastating. In the LEDCs, biomass fuels, and urban industry and transport are important sources of pollution and have serious consequences. In other parts of the world there are still similar problems. Pollution generated in low latitudes has even been noticed in remote parts of the Arctic.

12. Electro-magnetic fields generated by power lines and mobile phone masts has been associated with enhancing the effects of aerosol pollutants such as particles from traffic.

13. Farming practices in LEDCs have many adverse influences on the health of populations in those areas. Methods of increasing agricultural production can produce pesticide poisoning and the spread of irrigation encourages water-related diseases like malaria and schistosomiaisis (bilharzia). Food supplies are still an issue; famines will continue to threaten LEDCs, especially in Africa.

14. MEDC agriculture is divided over the effects of genetic modification (GM), which could enhance production methods, but could also pose a threat to the immune systems of plants, animals and even human populations.

15. Civil war and the consequent displacement of huge numbers of refugees leads to mortality on a very large scale. The lessons learned from the camps in Zaire after the Rwanda conflict will help to avoid such a large death toll in future.

16. Inadequate housing in MEDCs has many adverse effects on health, including asthma and lead poisoning. Rented housing in inner cities, especially linked with overcrowding, is detrimental to good health.

17. Crime can be linked to deprivation and poor environmental quality. Inner-city estates suffer from the fear of high rates of burglary and violence. Many aspects of the local environment such as housing design and poor lighting contribute to high crime rates.

18. Different races can have differing susceptibilities to diseases. The USA has an initiative which is designed to improve the health of all its ethnic groups.

Suggested essay or report title

Examine the ways in which the development and spread of infection follow geographical pathways and patterns.

As with all the suggested essay or report titles, it is the preparation (the research, in other words) which is just as important as the actual writing, if not more so.

Choice of title

- The title needs careful thought. Identify the command word. In this case it asks you to *examine*, which means '*to look in detail at*'.
- *Development* and *spread* are two different aspects of disease transmission. Also look at *pathways* (which suggests linear features such as rivers or roads or maybe airline routes) and *patterns* (which suggests clustering, random or equally spaced features which could have underlying human or physical causes such as settlement patterns or climate zones). These pathways and patterns can be static, or moving over time and space. Refer to these ideas at the start of the essay or report.

- Types of infectious disease and theories such as Kilbourne's waves, Bartlett's threshold theory, the Hamer–Sople island theory, Hagerstrand's diffusion theory, and core and periphery will be needed next. They should help you to explain the title in some way by relating it to what they would predict. It is just as valid to find situations where the theory does not hold true, as long as you can attempt to give *geographical* reasons for this.

Research

- The chart (frontispiece I) showing the outline of this chapter should give you some initial clues about how to answer a question on this generalisation. Make a large copy on A3 paper to act as a basic plan for your research and then add your own ideas and case studies from other sources to it.
- At this stage collect a good spread of relevant information.
- Be clear about the theoretical background to the essay or report.
- Remember to cover a good range of case studies.
- Be sure to make a full note of the sources of your information as a separate list.
- Include definitions of all the key words in the title: *infection, geographical pathway, geographical patterns.*

Planning

- The way in which you introduce each section of the essay or report is crucial. So, at this point, you should be numbering the topics (and the case studies which illustrate them) in a sequence which makes sense.
- One approach might be to look at
  - **Physical pathways**, taking (polluted) rivers such as the sewage-polluted Vistula in Poland or the fast-flowing rivers of West Africa which harbour the blackfly, vector of river blindness. **Physical patterns** might well relate to climates or biomes which allow infectious diseases or their vectors to flourish, such as the tsetse fly (sleeping sickness) or the anopheles mosquito (malaria).

  And then go on to

  - **Human pathways**, which can be transport routes; two options are the changing influences of mode of transport for speed of cholera transmission or the likelihood of measles being transmitted. **Human patterns** involve settlements, so the influenza epidemic charted in Northern England illustrating diffusion and core and periphery is useful. Refugees (such as those in Rwanda, Cambodia or Afghanistan, for instance) can be subject to all manner of infections in their pattern of enforced migration to temporary camps.

- If you want to put in a lot of information for case studies, annotated maps or spider diagrams are both excellent ways of summarising this.

Writing

- For the UK Edexcel B syllabus, your essay or report must be not more than 1,500 words long. It must show a clear sequence of ideas which are closely linked to what the question is demanding.

- A report must be written in a particular style, with headings, numbered sections and bullet points.
- It must have a report-style executive summary, no more than 10 sentences, describing the key contents, using technical terms and definitions, and setting the case studies in context. The summaries at the end of each chapter provide a guide to the style.
- The introduction must focus on the question and outline the direction the essay will take in attempting to answer it. It must justify your choice of case studies and link them to the theories which you want to use.
- Each paragraph must deal with a separate issue. The first sentence is like the 'headline' in a news report. The rest of the paragraph enlarges on the topic.
- Every idea or general statement should be backed up with evidence.
- Geographical terms show that your ideas are clear. You will be writing in a language which the examiner understands, and expects.
- It is pointless using maps and diagrams unless they are referred to in the text as a part of your evidenced discussion.
- An essay or report without a conclusion is like a sandwich without the bottom piece of bread. It is messy and difficult to digest.
- A conclusion sums up what you have discussed and evaluates just how far you agree with the question. It links theory with case studies to do this.
- The idea of 'lifting' large chunks of seemingly attractive text from sources such as the Internet is the wrong idea. It will have the wrong style and the wrong emphasis. All source material must be mentioned in the bibliography. This should tabulate each source, with its view or bias and a brief evaluation of how extreme this bias happens to be.

How does geography explain spatial variations in health and welfare patterns?

1 The epidemiological transition

a) What is the epidemiological transition?

When countries round the corner in the curve relating health to income, they also go through the so-called 'epidemiological transition'. The term is used to (mark) the change from predominantly infectious diseases, still common in poor countries, to the degenerative diseases, which have become the predominant cause of death in richer countries.

Richard G. Wilkinson, *Unhealthy Societies*, 1996

The trends shown in Figure 3.1a follow a pattern of change that seems to have taken about a century. When it has occurred in a particular country it seems to show that the bulk of the population has achieved a standard of living that provides all the basic necessities. Wilkinson calls this a '**minimum material standard**'. Thus great pandemics and famines will no longer pose the same threat and life expectancy will rise.

Related to this is a model suggested by Omran in 1971 (Figure 3.1b). Here it is clear that the types of diseases change through each stage. This has links with the Demographic Transition model, which traces the growth of a population, moving from very high to very low birth and mortality rates. Although both types of diseases are present throughout, the emphasis clearly changes as time progresses.

The original model had three stages. As populations in the developed world are ageing rapidly, a fourth stage has been added, with increased life expectancy. This is at the expense of poorer health in old age, as **delayed degenerative diseases** (such as prostate cancer, osteoporosis or Alzheimer's disease) become more common.

Infectious diseases are far from eliminated, however. The growth of HIV/AIDS in all societies, the threat of the so-called **re-emergent diseases** like MRSA and drug-resistant TB and the possibility of the northwards spread of tropical diseases with increased global warming, all suggest that they will continue to be important (see Chapter 5).

b) How is the epidemiological transition related to the global economy?

There are three ways in which Omran linked the epidemiological transition with patterns of economic growth :

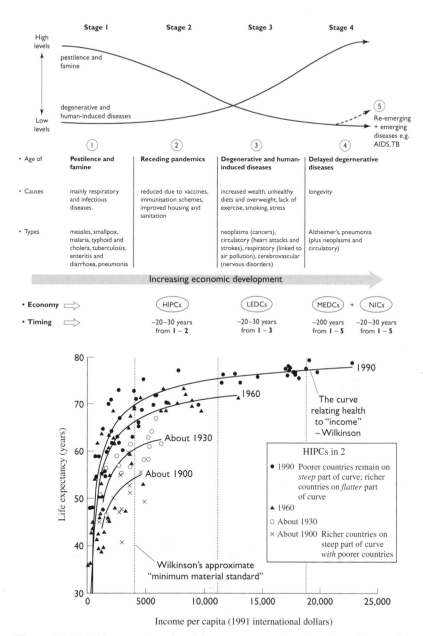

Figure 3.1 **a) Life expectancy and income per capita for selected countries and periods**
(Source: Wilkinson, R., *Unhealthy Societies*, Routledge 1996)
b) The epidemiological transition after Omran 1971

1. **The 'western' countries pattern followed by the MEDCs**. This has taken over a century to move through stages one to four.
2. **The 'accelerated' change**, which has happened in most NICs.
3. **The 'delayed' change in LEDCs** with high fertility rates and infectious diseases still prominent but with an additional increase in degenerative diseases.

c) How far does this help to explain variations in health and welfare?

The epidemiological transition can be a useful way of interpreting health patterns and trends worldwide. However, the picture is more complex in reality:

- While a country might experience a rising GNP pc, there is no guarantee that any extra will go towards health spending. Other priorities, such as defence or debt servicing, might have prior claims on resources. If the state decides not take responsibility for health and welfare provision for the majority of its population, the relationship between GNP pc and life expectancy could be further weakened.
- Any investment in health taken from increasing national wealth must be targeted correctly. Numbers of health professionals may well have little influence on the health of a population in the early stages of the epidemiological transition. McKeown's (1975) studies of the UK (quoted by Wilkinson) demonstrate that the decline in mortality from infectious diseases owed far more to clean water supply, sanitation, shelter and nutrition than from any medical advances.
- It is significant that, in the late stages of the transition, those diseases that were once linked with affluence in the middle stages, such as coronary heart disease, stoke, high blood pressure and duodenal ulcers, become far more common in the less well off. This is particularly true of obesity, once regarded as an asset in those societies where famine was common.
- Once a country has reached stage four, the relationship between rising GNP pc and life expectancy levels off (Figure 3.1). According to Wilkinson, what causes any further rises in life expectancy is not continued economic growth but improvements in the equality of the provision.

2 Health and inequalities

a) How can inequalities be measured?

The measurement of inequalities is only as good as the data used in their calculation. Chapter 1 discusses the methods which can be used to measure them. Frequently this takes the form of a **composite index** using social, economic and even environmental indicators.

In the UK, the **four measures of deprivation**, outlined in Chapter 1, used to investigate health inequalities are:

1. The Jarman Index
2. The Carstairs Index
3. The Townsend Index
4. The DETR Index

These are often employed as a tool for future planning and broader social policy. The UK government's report 'Our Healthy Nation' in the early 1990s stimulated Health Authorities to examine the extent of health inequalities in their areas.

The Health of Londoners Project (a group of London Health Authorities) produced ' Deprivation and Health in London' in 1996. The particular factors influencing health in London were: the disproportionately high numbers of young people; a large transient population; areas with high material deprivation; great ethnic diversity; many vulnerable populations such as the homeless, refugees, those in poor housing, the unemployed and the elderly.

Poverty and deprivation figured largely in the analysis. The key issues were seen to be: infectious disease; sexual health; substance abuse; mental health; availability of primary care services.

Using the **Jarman Index** a fairly clear relationship between the level of deprivation and the SMR (standard mortality rate) from 1981 to 1991 emerged. Bromley, a favoured outer borough, had a score of −10, whereas the impoverished Tower Hamlets scored +72 during this period. Mortality rates in London in general fell less rapidly than in the UK overall between 1981 to 1991. Those of young men were 20% higher. Inner-city boroughs were the worst affected.

The Trent Area Health Authority made an extensive study in 1998, using the Townsend Index to highlight deficiencies (Figure 3.2). The region extends from the picturesque Peak District to the old Yorkshire, Nottinghamshire and Derby coalfield (with its declining heavy industries of mining, steel, engineering and textiles) and across rural Lincolnshire to the port of Grimsby on Humberside.

Mapping the **Townsend Index** for the Trent Area reveals strong contrasts (Figure 3.3). The main area showing deprivation (high positive scores) is associated with the industrial South Yorkshire conurbation. The more rural area to the east is less deprived. Even so, there are pockets of privilege in, for instance, south-west Sheffield (as urban models for the UK might predict). Looking at morbidity and mortality data for the area reinforces these links. The provision of health care follows a similar pattern.

In a report from 1996, Doncaster Health Authority used a Relative Needs Index (RNI) to assess General Practice provision. This was based on:

* levels of unemployment
* proportion of elderly people living alone
* proportion of single carer households
* proportion of people with limiting long-term illness.

Health Districts by Townsend Score, 1991. Trent Region		
	Health District	Townsend Score (Standardised to Trent Region)
DISADVANTAGE	Sheffield	4.81
	Barnsley	3.86
	Doncaster	3.28
	Rotherham	2.63
	Nottingham	0.72
	Southern Derbyshire	−1.18
	South Humber*	−1.71
	North Nottinghamshire	−2.98
	Leicestershire	−1.92
	North Derbyshire	−3.03
ADVANTAGE	Lincolnshire	−4.54

* South Humber is calculated combining Grimsby and Scunthorpe.

Figure 3.2 **Townsend Index Scores for Trent Region Health Districts 1991**
(Source: Trent Area Health Authority – Sheffield)

Relating the RNI to staffing of GPs and practice nurses shows far too low a level of expenditure in those practices with high need (Figure 3.4) There is a shortage of GPs in the South Yorkshire conurbation, with a deficit of:

- 38 in Rotherham
- 28 in Doncaster
- 21 in Barnsley.

The rural areas to east and west all show a slight surplus.

Other useful composite indices for health, used by the UNDP on a global scale, are the **Human Development Index (HDI)** and its related index, the **Gender-Related Development Index (GDI)**. These are calculated using national income, life expectancy, adult literacy and years in education. The GDI includes a measure of female advancement. The result measures national human progress (a total near to 1.0 is good; those nations with the smallest rates of advance score less than 0.1).

The World Bank uses **two measures of inequality** in its Highly Indebted Poor Countries (HIPC) health reports. The first is the **poor/rich ratio** (the ratio between the incomes of the top and bottom 20% of the population). The **concentration index** measures the concentration of different health variables across income groups. It varies from +1 to −1, with zero showing no concentration.

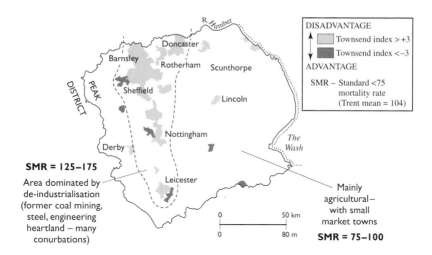

Figure 3.3 **Trent Area Health Authority map showing contrasting Townsend**
scores and main mortality differences
(Source: data from (ibid))

It is generally agreed that of all the single economic and social indicators (for example, GDP pc and number of doctors per patient
respectively) the most accurate picture of a country's health is given
by the **Infant Mortality rate (IMR/1,000 live births)** or, even better,
the **U5 IMR (under-five IMR)**. The reasoning is that any nation
should value its new population most highly. This emphasises the
importance of caring for pregnant women and, ultimately, for their
vulnerable offspring. This should be a key resource target for all societies. Consequently, these mortality rates figure strongly in any discussion of inequality measurement.

b) Why should Richard Wilkinson say that 'inequality kills'?

The causes and consequences of inequalities in health are the subject
of heated debate. Since **social policy** (state provision) is often
directed by research in this field, understanding the issues involved is
an important part of the study of health and welfare.

The two sides of the argument are introduced below:

Health is telling us a story about the major influences on quality of life in modern societies – a story we cannot afford to
ignore ...qualitative change is more important than quantitative
growth ...What affects health is no longer the differences in
absolute material standards, but social position within societies.

Richard G. Wilkinson, op. cit

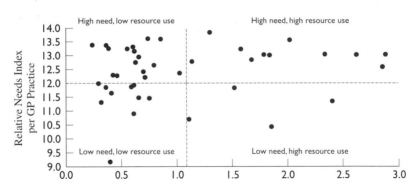

Number of staff (GPs and practice nurses) per 1000 GP Practice population

Figure 3.4 **Relationship between Relative Needs Index and number of GPs with their employed staff, by GP practice 1996, Doncaster**
(Source: (ibid))

The benevolent evolutionary view of the epidemiological transition from mainly infectious to chronic diseases, which underlies models of social cohesion and social capital, has been used to justify the shift from material to psycho-social causes of health inequalities...which is not warranted.

J. Lynch, *Journal of Epidemiology and Community Medicine*, 2000

Wilkinson's main ideas may be summarised as follows:

1. Overall health standards in population groups and societies, rather than in individuals, are important.
2. Health seems to be a better guide to quality of life than GNP pc or real income measures.
3. Health inequalities within societies are mostly a reflection of the social and economic circumstances of different groups in society, rather than being related to genetics, medical care or lifestyle.
4. The relative differences in standards of living within MEDCs, not between them, can explain variations in mortality rates. In other words, it is **relative poverty** (what each individual lacks in relation to the more fortunate in a society; often taken as below half the average income in the UK) which determines health status. **Absolute poverty** (the lack of the basic necessities for life, for instance, food, shelter, clean water and security) has less effect on the population as economic growth advances.
5. **Social cohesion** – a strong community network characterised by lively involvement and concern for others (sometimes called **social capital**) creates a healthy society in every meaning of the word.
6. In countries and societies which are inegalitarian (with great inequalities and therefore showing **social disintegration**) there is a greater degree of social stress which leads to increased crime, violence and homicide.

7. Societies suffering **social disintegration**, in turn, have higher mortality rates among the under-fives (U5 IMR).
8. The **psycho-social influences** on health are more important than any others, once the country is in the later stages of the epidemiological transition.
9. Positive psycho-social factors include active social networks and community involvement and a taller population (as increased height can indicate having avoided stress when growing during childhood and a greater emotional stability).
10. Negative psycho-social factors include insecurity over housing, employment and debts leading to chronic stress.
11. In short, as mortality rates of societies with higher rates of inequalities are shown to be higher; 'inequality kills'.

Wilkinson gives instances where this is the case:

• In the UK during the two world wars, where income differences were levelled out as everyone endured shortages, people's health improved. Life expectancy rose (from 1.2 years more than in 1900 in 1931–40 to 6.5 years more than in 1900 in 1941–50).
• In the small town of Roseto, Pennsylvania, in 1950, most of the population was descended from the original Italian settlers who had arrived some 80 years before. The only difference from other towns in the area seemed to be its strong community spirit and the classless nature of the society. At that time, the mortality rates from cardiovascular disease were 40% less than those of its neighbours. Once outside influences arrived in the 1960s, the community became less well-knit and its health advantage was lost.
• In post-war Japan, industry became far more democratic, with little demarcation between workers and management. The companies were, in effect, a welfare state and an extended family for their employees. Life expectancy in Japan rose to be one of the highest in the world, although economic downturn has altered the picture a little.

Lynch's (2000) point is that the so-called **'buffering hypothesis'** (which maintains that denser social support networks create better health in a community by protecting against stress) is only part of the picture. The improvements in **material standards of living** (for instance, better insulated houses, improved access to medical care, awareness of the importance of exercise and a well-balanced diet) also have a part to play in increasing life expectancy. The continuing drop in mortality rates from cardiovascular disease in New Zealand, the UK and Finland bears this out. Lynch likens this effect to that of the social improvements in the UK in the nineteenth century.

Whatever the essential factors behind these inequalities, all agree that they should be reduced. Woodward (2000) suggests why this should be done:

- they are, above all, unfair and unjust
- some types of inequality have a 'spill-over effect' on the whole of society, such as alcohol and drug abuse, the spread of infectious diseases (HIV/AIDS, TB) or violence and crime
- government action (social policy) can help by providing tax benefits and health and welfare funding
- any programmes introduced are usually cost-effective (cervical screening to prevent cancer, for instance).

Work done by Chiang (2000) in Taiwan provides a clear picture of a rapidly developing NIC and the consequent changes to patterns of life expectancy and mortality rates in relation to income distribution. The country changed from a predominantly agricultural import-orientated economy in 1953, when the GNP pc was $196, to an industrialised export-based one in 1995, with a GNP pc of $12,396. During this time, the income distribution became increasingly favourable. At the beginning, the poor/rich ratio was 20. By 1995, the figure was only 5. The graphs (Figure 3.5) show the remarkable effects this had on life expectancy and mortality rates. These results agree closely with Wilkinson's ideas. However, Taiwan is only one case and the combination of increasing equality and rapid economic growth is an unusual occurrence.

Hales (2000) used data from the World Bank for 1970 and 1990 to investigate the relationship between IMR, GNP pc and income inequality in 38 countries. It was found that in those poor countries (< $1,000 GNP pc) where income inequalities were reduced or where GNP pc went up, IMR rates showed a reduction. In richer countries, reduction of income inequalities had a greater effect on IMR than an increase in GNP pc.

c) Do health indicators follow the core and periphery model?

In order to relate health indicators to Friedmann's core-periphery model (which suggests that certain core areas have a concentration of population, wealth and resources and that the periphery is less developed), it is necessary to look at a variety of scales. The variation within and between areas is also worth noting:

- On a local scale, such as in a city like London, the deprived inner areas with poor health indicators, especially those on the eastern side (following urban models such as Mann's) contrast markedly with the more prosperous outer suburbs. The periphery here is favoured, not disadvantaged.
- On a regional scale (see Figure 3.3), the old industrial core region of South Yorkshire is again a focal point for poor deprivation scores and consequent ill health while the rural areas are better.
- Nationally, in England, there is a general trend towards lower rates for

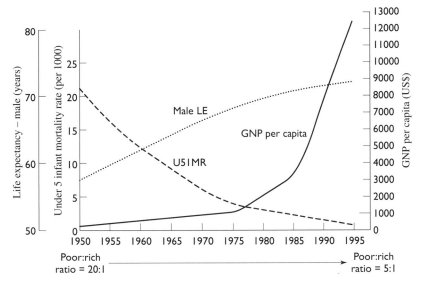

Figure 3.5 **Graph plotting male life expectancy and under five
mortality rate against GNP pc – Taiwan 1953–95
(after Chiang 2000)**
(Source: data from Chiang 2000 BMJ 319 (7218): 1162)

the prosperous south and east as far as life expectancy is concerned. This
is revealed by Soni Raleigh and Kiri (1997) in their study of longevity. In
1996, Cambridge and Dorset seemed to have the highest life expectan-
cies for both men and women (76.6 years and 81.4 years respectively
against national means of 74.1 and 79.5). The gap between these figures
and those for the deprived northern inner cities such as Manchester and
Liverpool had increased markedly from 4.2 years for men and 4.2 years
for women in 1984 to 5.2 years for men and 4.7 years for women in
1996. The five authorities with the lowest male life expectancy have, not
unsurprisingly, the lowest Jarman scores.

- On a continental scale, the WHO report on Health in Europe in the late
  1990s compares the prosperous regions of Western Europe with the
  newly independent states of the Confederation of Independent States
  (CIS) of the former Soviet Bloc. Life expectancy at birth is 11 years
  greater in the West. In the East it actually declined from 73.1 to 72.4
  years from 1991 to 1994.
- The main global division is the North–South divide, as defined by the
  Brandt commission in 1980. This is reinforced by the Development Gap
  model described in the Human Development Report 1994. The MEDCs,
  naturally, have the concentration of wealth and resources that enables
  them to achieve an impressive range of health scores. Around 85% of
  global income is from the richest 20% of countries. The bottom 20%,

poor LEDCs – known as HIPCs (Highly Indebted Poor Countries) by the World Bank – produce under 2% of global GNP.

The WHO report for 2000 lists life expectancy for 191 countries:

- Japan is top of the list, with 77.6 years for men and 84.3 years for women.
- The Russian Foundation (a former planned economy) is 91st with 62.7 and 74.0 years respectively. The collapse of the communist system in 1990 and the subsequent chaos brought worsening health services to all but the very rich (see Chapter 5).
- At the bottom of the list is Sierra Leone, which has been ravaged by war, international debt, food shortages and now a terrifyingly rapid spread of AIDS/HIV infection. Here the life expectancy for men is only an appalling 33.3 years and for women, only 35.4 years.

These figures correspond well to the Human Development Index (HDI) rankings proposed by the UN Development Programme in 1990. This uses per capita real income and adult literacy levels in addition to life expectancy.

d) What did the WHO league table 2000 show?

The World Health Organisation produces annual reports on different aspects of global health each year. The World Health Report 2000 concentrated on assessing the performance of national health systems. As the Director-General, Gro Harlem Brundtland, points out:

> the main message from this report is that the health and well-being of people around the world depend critically on the performance of the health systems that serve them. Yet there is wide variation in performance, even among countries with similar levels of income and health expenditure. It is essential for decision-makers to understand the underlying reasons so that health system performance, and hence the health of populations, can be improved.

Any failures in health systems have their greatest impact on the poor. 'They are treated with less respect, given less choice of service providers and offered lower-quality amenities. In trying to buy health from their own pockets, they pay and become poorer.'

The assessment of health systems was based on five indicators:

1. overall levels of population health (using a measure of life expectancy in relation to an estimation of the years affected by disability at the end of life – DALE or Disability Adjusted Life Expectancy)
2. health inequalities (disparities) within the population
3. overall level of health system responsiveness (combining patient satisfaction and how well the health system performs)

4. how people of varying economic status find that they are served by the health system
5. who pays for health costs.

The general trend is shown in which plots performance against health expenditure pc. The global variations that emerged led to France being top of the list of 191 countries. Other European countries which rated highly were Italy 2nd, Spain 7th and Norway 11th. The UK came 18th. Latin American countries Columbia and Chile came 22nd and 33rd respectively. Singapore is ranked 6th and Japan 10th. New Zealand ranks 32nd, with Australia 41st. Middle Eastern countries did well. Oman had very a high IMR in 1970 but ranked 8th overall in 2000, showing how impressive its government's efforts to improve healthcare have been.

3 Julian Tudor Hart and the Inverse Care Law

a) What is the Inverse Care Law?

The graph (Figure 3.6a) shows the situation of **inverse care**. Where there is great need, there is little expenditure on healthcare. Hence the logical solution is turned upside down or **inverted**. It is important to distinguish, however, between **need** for services and **demand** for them (Meade & Earickson 2000). The need for a qualified doctor by those who are ill is a necessity, but there may be the demand for plastic surgery even though it is usually a luxury. If all areas were to be equally well served then the situation known as **territorial justice** would exist. The graph (Figure 3.6b) shows that need is balanced equally at any

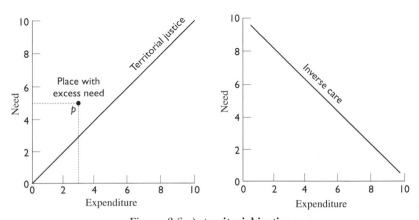

Figure 3.6 **a) territorial justice**
b) inverse care
(Source: in Meade & Earickson Medical Geography Guilford Press 2000)

expenditure level. The needs of the population, represented by point p on the graph, show **inequality** because they are not all being met.

Julian Tudor Hart was a doctor working in South Wales. In the light of his experiences there, he wrote an article for the medical journal, *The Lancet*, in 1971. In it he stated his **Inverse Care Law**:

the availability of good medical care tends to vary inversely with the need for it in the population served.

The richer areas, he noted, were well served with doctors both in the community and in hospitals, but the poor, who, especially in a mining area like South Wales, had greater need of medical support were not. This seemed illogical and discriminatory, to say the least.

b) What geographical factors influence it?

The reasons he gave for his observation were as follows:

* Industrial and mining areas tended to lack hospital medicine provision, even though they were served by GPs.
* The GPs were often in single-handed practices, which made it difficult to offer a high quality service at all times.
* Most medical professionals, having sufficient resources to do so, preferred to live in pleasant residential areas which did not suffer from the problems associated with deprivation; Few actively sought out the poorer areas.

The findings for Trent (Figures 3.2, 3.3 and 3.4) and London show that this is certainly true for impoverished inner cities and 'rust belt' industrial and mining areas in the UK.

In those countries with little state health provision, where insurance schemes do not cover the poorer workers (such as the USA) or in many LEDCs, where direct payments are made for health services (such as India), good medical care is lacking for those who need it most (see Chapter 5). In the USA, 40 million people on low wages have limited access to healthcare, using under-resourced 'Welfare' hospitals where accident and emergency waiting times can run to 15 hours. In India, families typically have to pay 80% of their healthcare costs, which means that many would simply not be able to seek assistance from other than a local 'traditional' healer without getting far into debt.

In Pakistan, Karachi, with a population of well over 12 million, has two hospitals which provide stark contrasts, according to McCormick and Fisher-Hoch (1996):

The Civil Hospital has the desolate look of a skeleton with a few rags hung on it ...the hospital has deteriorated markedly over the last several years ...because of a system that allows doctors to reach the most prestigious posts because of favouritism and connections . . .medical schools assign little importance to family medicine . . . .The hospital is the medical facility of last resort for thousands of residents. They are united by their need for urgent medical care – and by their poverty . . .the sad fact is that they are required to purchase most of the medicines and supplies they need. This 1,700-bed hospital is the largest in the country. Typhoid and cholera account for a large number of patients.

It would be difficult to find a more dramatic contrast between the Civil Hospital and the hospital at Aga Khan University (AKU), located in a fashionable suburb . . .one of the best facilities of its kind . . .it was built of marble, tile and stucco ten years ago at . . .the stupendous cost of $300 million . . .for the most part, the hospital is available to the relatively more wealthy; there is no medical insurance to speak of. The red sandstone walls of the building use a traditional desert design, which creates constant shadow . . .Nevertheless, AKU is struggling with how to provide excellent health services to all, including the poor, and pay for it. It is a social-economic schizophrenia, for which there is no easy cure.

c) Can it be remedied?

Using a tool such as the Lorenz Curve (Figure 3.7), the **distribution** of healthcare services over an area can be analysed. Uniform Care (compare Figure 3.6b) will have a straight line. On a curve to show the actual pattern in an area to compare with this, **clustering** will show a gentler gradient, whereas a more **uniform** pattern will steepen the line.

The Gini Index (see Figure 3.7),. which shows the difference between a perfectly even distribution of healthcare resources and reality, can also quantify the problem for healthcare providers.

Central place theory, a model first described by Christaller in the 1930s, states that the quantity and variety of goods and services available to a given population vary with the number of people who have access to theses goods and services. Cities are at the top of a hierarchy (a structured arrangement) in offering a wide range, including **high-order services** (such as MRI body scanners and open heart surgery). Smaller settlements offer only those **lower-order services**, which are profitable with fewer consumers (such as minor operations or first aid treatment). In the model the larger settlements are further apart.

Counteracting the Inverse Care Law could be as simple as organising the health service according to the hierarchy of central place theory so that there was an even spread of facilities and of personnel throughout the country. Knox's work in the early 1970s in Edinburgh shows that middle-class areas have a more accessible primary care (GP) service than do peripheral 'deprived' estates. In the former Soviet Union there was indeed a lavish provision of resources and

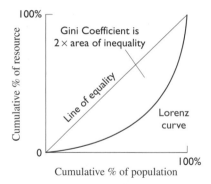

Figure 3.7 **A Lorenz Curve and generalised Gini Index**
(Source: in (ibid))

these were evenly spaced, but there was no control over outcomes (see Chapter 5). All new doctors were required to work first in rural areas, guaranteeing country people healthcare. The new system has no such restrictions and many doctors have left for the cities (Ensor 1995). The Chinese system was also based on a hierarchy, but rising incomes have led to its collapse in rural areas (see Chapter 5). Only Cuba – still a communist state – conforms to the pattern (see Chapter 5).

Even if there *are* healthcare facilities, they might be as detrimental to health as those in Zaire (now the Democratic Republic of the Congo) where Ebola virus was spread through poor hygiene (see Chapter 4). They could also be staffed by incompetent doctors, as in Sierra Leone (see Chapter 5).

4 How does socio-economic status influence access to healthcare?

Those groups in society that are vulnerable to poor health, for whatever reason, are often denied proper access to health and welfare services, as Tudor Hart found. Often they lack either the information, resources, or power to improve their situation. They are usually those at the bottom of the inequality 'heap' and subject to the 'poverty cycle', where one difficulty reinforces another. It is quite possible for an individual to belong to more than one category of those listed below, in which case the problem is compounded still further.

a) The poor

In the UK

> Poverty is a principal source of ill health. Poor people are ill more often and die sooner.
>
> Frank Dobson, Secretary of State for Health, November 1998

Narrowing the gap between rich and poor could prevent as many as 10,000 premature deaths each year in Britain, according to a report published by the Joseph Rowntree Foundation yesterday. Even a modest redistribution of wealth and income, restoring inequalities to their 1983 levels, would save 7,500 under-65s a year.

The Times, 26 September 2000

From the mid-1980s to the mid-1990s, the number of people in the UK living in relative poverty increased markedly. In 1996 a survey by health visitors found that one in three British babies was born into poverty. Malnutrition, poor living conditions, fuel debt and electricity and gas disconnections were particular problems. One response to this was Sir Donald Acheson's Report of the Independent Enquiry into Inequalities in Health in 1998. This identified as many as 39 strategies to improve the health of the poor, such as:

- higher benefits and pensions
- free nicotine patches
- school meals and fresh fruit
- fluoridation
- better housing.

Commenting on these, the Royal College of General Practitioners was careful to point out that increasing resources allocated to a specific health problem did not always reach those who needed it most. People in deprived areas often have little systematic healthcare (such as regular dental checks) and low levels of preventive care (such as childhood immunisations). Social problems in a practice overstretch the medical professionals too. Patients from poor areas *do* visit the GP frequently, but often about accidents and infectious diseases rather than about preventive care. Poorer people are more likely to develop cancer, associated with increased smoking in some cases, but are less likely to seek help until the symptoms are more advanced. Giving deprivation payments to inner-city GPs cannot solve all the problems, as motivating GPs to see the positive side of working in inner cities is difficult.

From 1999–2002, as a part of the UK government's 'Our Healthier Nation' initiative, £290 million will be put into 26 Health Action Zones (HAZs). These have the aims of:

- improving health
- tackling inequalities
- modernising services.

They represent multi-agency partnerships with the NHS, running for seven years. Most are based in the northern industrial cities and in inner London.

In Central and Eastern Europe

The WHO report on European Health in 1997 identified a growing percentage of the European population living in poverty. Related to low income was inadequate diet and, as a consequence, disease. Many people on fixed incomes spent up to 75% of their disposable income on food, leaving little for other health needs. Most of the problems have emerged in the CIS (newly independent states of the former Soviet Union) and in CCEE (central and eastern Europe, formerly communist). In these areas the real value of wages began to fall rapidly in 1989. The pressures on the welfare state systems in Western Europe were also growing, but not as dramatically. Reforming the provision of healthcare in the NIS and in the CCEE from a centrally planned to an insurance system has been slow and inefficient, with the selection of the more prosperous, healthier population for insurance rather than the poor (obviously those in poorer health). This practice is known as 'cherry picking'. Thus the poor are socially marginalised.

Bobak (1998) reinforces the idea of the gradient between poverty and plenty as being an important factor in health.

There is evidence from European countries of inequity in access to good quality medical care. This will exacerbate the problems of inequalities in health …One way of thinking about medical care is that it is part of **social capital**. Access to good quality, humane and cost-effective medical care is a necessary feature of a civilised society.

Not only health professionals but also medicines are hard to find for the poor. Anna Blundy, writing about the Russian Federation (see Chapter 5) in *The Times* in 2000 comments:

there is a terrible shortage of basic medicines and what is available is often imported and increasingly expensive. There are now chemists in Moscow whose pharmacies do not look a lot worse than Boots, but a packet of Nurofen would clean out the average monthly pension and the number of people who can afford the imported prescriptions is vanishing into insignificance …clinics in Moscow catering for Westerners and very rich Russians …all ask how you are paying before they ask how you are …

In the USA

In the USA, those on welfare support receive healthcare help from the Medicaid system as do those over 65 from Medicare (see Chapter 5). However, there is a growing number of people – over 40 million – on low wages, who cannot afford the health insurance they need for themselves and their children. The implications are that they are not only reluctant to seek medical help, but are also unlikely to have used preventive care (screening or immunisation). There are schemes to help. Around 80% of those insured indicated their willingness to subsidise the 'uninsured' in taxes by extending Medicaid and the Children's Health Insurance Program (CHIP). Most uninsured would have to give up basic necessities such as food rent and utility bills in order to buy health insurance. In a survey in 2000, 30% of the uninsured reported that they had been in debt in the previous year.

In Indiana State one in seven adults are uninsured (70,000 people). One reason is that the economic upturn in the 1990s meant more employment, but many of the low-paid jobs did not come with health insurance 'packages'. In response to the CHIP initiative offering states $24 billion over five years, Indiana set up 500 enrolment centres for their Hoosier Healthwise program so that children could be supported. Nearly 200,000 children were signed up in the first two years.

In LEDCs

Extreme inequalities in most of the developing world mean that the task of helping the poor to gain access to healthcare is an enormous one. One way forward is the provision of basic improvements in health and hygiene education. Measures like these go towards reducing the incidence of some of the main killer diseases such as diarrhoea. These initial steps are more important than improving medical provision alone, especially as many rural people find themselves several days' walk from the nearest hospital or doctor and with few resources to pay fees for treatment or for drugs in any case.

One NGO with long experience in this field is Oxfam, which 'never stops striving to find better ways to combat poverty and to help poor people to make lasting improvements to their lives'.

- Recent Oxfam initiatives include the 'Oxfam Bucket', introduced in 1997. This has a tight-fitting cover and an integral cap. Collecting and storing drinking water is made safer, especially in emergency situations for the poor in conflicts such as those in Mozambique and Angola.
- In Sierra Leone, refugees are taught by Oxfam-trained Hygiene promoters, who are refugees themselves. Basic hygiene is helped by the use of an Oxfam bucket, scrubbing brush, soap and a measuring jug for Oral Re-hydration Therapy (ORT), a simple but effective way of fighting diarrhoea.
- In northern Ghana, the provision of just one motor bike made it possible for a medical assistant from Oxfam to reach 25,000 people in 30 remote villages in order to give regular vaccinations and health information.

In Nepal there are only around 300 physicians serving a population of over 6 million. But there are 400,000 traditional rural healers. They do not show in official figures, but they have basic health training and sell essential medical products to the rural poor. They are in daily contact with the rural people and understand popular culture. They are very useful in suggesting ways of promoting large-scale health promotion programmes in collaboration with UNICEF, for example. Combining the sale of ORT salts, as diarrhoea treatment, with exorcism of evil spirits is common.

b) Women and childbirth

No society treats its women as well as its men.

UNDP Human development report, 1997.

Many women have lower income and lower social standing than men and often lack education, but now they are marrying later and are having fewer children. The effects of the spread of female education have been to improve the health of both mothers and the whole family. **Female life expectancy** has increased from 71.0 to 74.6 in MEDCs and from 54.5 to 62.4 in LEDCs. However, in spite of falling birth rates worldwide (the **fertility rate** – mean number of births per woman – in Thailand has gone down from 6.4 in 1963 to 2.1 in 1993, in Tunisia from 7.1 to 3.1, in Kuwait from 7.3 to 3.1, and in Brazil from 6.1 to 2.9) women are still at risk through pregnancy and childbirth.

Maternal mortality is up to 50 times higher in LEDCs than in the developed world. More than 500,000 women die each year as a result of pregnancy and childbirth, almost all in LEDCs. The 1 million motherless children left behind will themselves have reduced life expectancy. All these deaths could be prevented with access to basic reproductive healthcare. The maternal mortality rate in Sierra Leone is one in seven women. **Perinatal mortality** is also high, with 50 infants per 100,000 live births dying in Sierra Leone.

Projects seeking to redress the balance include:
* Save the Children working in Bangladesh with UJON, a local charity, to improve antenatal care in the spontaneous settlements around Khulna, where 30,000 people live. The project began in 1995, preventing still births by helping with nutritional programmes and running a credit and savings scheme to help small businesses.
* Young female prostitutes in Recife, in Brazil, are being given help through a day centre which provides education, medical attention and health advice, especially if they become pregnant.

Even in MEDCs, reduced access to healthcare is associated with low birthweight babies. McLafferty and Tempalski have shown the clear relationship between the spatial distribution of low birthweight babies (less than 2.5 kilograms), clinics and women below the poverty line in New York City. The rise in low birthweight babies reflected areas where women's falling social status and low insurance levels were linked to high crack cocaine abuse. Many were 3 or 4 kilometres from the nearest clinic.

Male children are preferred, partly for religious reasons. The incidence of **infanticide** (child murder) and deliberate starvation among girl babies is high in some areas, often owing to the perceived problems of financing a dowry (marriage settlement) in later life. About 16 million baby girls a year are killed by their mothers or by village midwives in Tamil Nadu state, Southern India. This affects only the lower classes, as they do not have enough to provide for their children and cannot afford tests to establish the sex of a baby during pregnancy and subsequent abortions. The first daughter is allowed to live as she can help with household chores. Any further girls are not, as they are too expensive to marry off. Grooms can expect a dowry of around 25,000 rupees (£500), 100 grams of gold, household goods and a car before they contemplate marriage. In most countries there are 105 women to every 100 men. In Tamil Nadu the ratio is 93:100. In China it is 88:100, also due to female infanticide and the One Child population control policy.

In many societies where **contraception** is expensive or difficult to find, abortion becomes an important method of family planning. This is a leading cause of maternal mortality in itself. In the Russian Federation, falling living standards and rapid contraceptive price rises have led to a higher rate of unwanted pregnancies. **Abortion** is free on demand up to 22 weeks of pregnancy for reasons such as cramped living conditions. In 1992, 3.5 million abortions were performed. In 1997, the figure was 2.5 million, but there were only 1.25 million live births (Marcus Warren, *Sunday Telegraph*, 1999). The effects have been disastrous. Nearly 40% of the operations result in complications needing expensive drugs or hospital treatment, which many cannot afford. One in eight couples is now infertile. Lack of condoms raises the risk of sexually transmitted disease. The population is dropping at the rate of around 500,000 a year. The Orthodox Church is attempting to reverse the trend, but is seriously underfunded.

UNICEF maintains that if four basic interventions were to be introduced, the majority of maternal deaths and about half of all the infant deaths and maternal disabilities could be prevented. The interventions are:

1. improved access to basic health, family planning services and adequate nutrition
2. attendance at birth by either a skilled midwife or a doctor
3. essential obstetric care for complications and emergencies
4. post-natal and basic neo-natal care.

The cost is estimated at around £1.60 per person per year for those at risk. There is no real need for hundreds more hospitals and thousands more expensively trained obstetricians.

c) Homelessness

Even in MEDCs, such as the UK, homelessness is a significant problem. In 1999 there were an estimated 400,000 homeless people. Of these, 78,000 were couples or lone parents sharing accommodation as they could not afford a home of their own, 41,000 were living in hostels or squats and 1,600 were on the streets. In addition to this were the 'unofficially' homeless who do not generally seek help from the authorities. Some estimates suggest that there are over 1 million of them, mainly single homeless people.

The reasons why people become homeless often lie in family conflict. Around 25% of homeless families were without somewhere to live because of a relationship breakdown. Many of these had been forced to move owing to physical abuse. Children suffer particularly; 60% of homeless families have dependent children.

The effects of homelessness on health are many. Families, crammed into women's refuges, fleeing from violent relationships, or sharing inadequate bed-and-breakfast accommodation in run-down hotels, lead unhealthy lives. Overcrowding leads to the rapid spread of infection and the children have low rates of immunisation because of their frequent moves. Cooking facilities are poor and a balanced diet is virtually impossible on a low income.

Single people fare worse. Even if they use night hostels or shelters they suffer from the cold, they are dirty and are inadequately nourished. The hostels are full and alcohol abuse is rife. Mortality rates are often 25 times higher than in the population as a whole. Many suffer from bronchitis and pneumonia. The incidence of TB is 200 times the mean UK rate; 2% of the single homeless suffer from TB. Life on the streets compounds these problems: respiratory diseases flourish, foot and muscle complaints worsen and skin ulcers grow. Accidents and mental illness are all too common.

Despite all these problems, the homeless have poor access to healthcare. GPs can be reluctant to register individuals with no fixed address (although one local authority recently allowed a group of single homeless to give their 'home' as a particular park bench to allow them to receive post and essential medical and welfare benefits!). Owing to frequent moves, many homeless people experience no continuity in their medical care. Accident and emergency departments in hospitals are frequently used by homeless people for primary care which should be given by a GP. It is estimated that 57% of visits to A and E departments by the homeless are 'inappropriate'. In South London, a programme of mass X-ray screening of hostel dwellers for TB incidence actually took the equipment to the hostels. In spite of this positive move, however, only 14% of those whose tests needed following up actually kept their appointments. (Stevens 1992)

At the other extreme, those made homeless through war, conflict and disaster in LEDCs suffer greatly. Frequently they are housed at best in makeshift camps where even the most basic provision of clean water, shelter and sanitation is scarce or altogether absent. Being subject to climatic extremes, in addition, puts them in a near impossible situation.

In a remote highland area in the east of Cambodia some 30,000 people, many of whom are refugees returned from Thailand, are suffering from extreme food shortages and virtually no social services, education or medical care. In 2000, Refugees International, a US NGO, assisted in putting more land into cultivation for shifting agriculture. Also needed were disease prevention for malaria and other serious tropical diseases, and far more equipment for the provincial hospital, which severely lacked staff and supplies. Medecins du Monde, a French NGO, was the only body attempting to provide clinics, immunisations and public health assistance in the area.

d) Drug users

The misuse of alcohol and tobacco, in addition to illegal drugs like cannabis, opiates and amphetamines, accounts for a significant percentage of health problems. Their users are often caught in a vicious spiral of decline but their habits themselves make it difficult to reverse the trend. Often the drugs seem to offer an escape from difficult circumstances, but in reality they make the situation worse.

An area where drug abuse of all kinds has reached alarming proportions is in the former Soviet Union and its satellites (now the CCEE and CIS)

- Major differences in life expectancy between the CCEE (central and eastern Europe) and the CIS (newly independent states, formerly the Soviet Union) have become apparent in the 1990s. The main reason seems to be in drinking habits. Excessive drinking of vodka and brandy was common until 1985 in the old Soviet Union, when there was a severe restriction in the sale of alcohol. This led to a sharp drop in fatal accidents, suicides and homicides. After 1991, however, with a market economy, alcohol, often produced illegally, was available at very low prices. By 1994 the mortality rate was even higher than it had been before 1985. This was also associated with deaths from sudden heart failure brought about from binge drinking in men aged between 25 and 65. Chronic alcoholics referred to clinics for treatment rose to 50 per 100,000 of the population and were mainly male.
- Smoking prevalence surveys conducted in Moscow and St Petersburg showed that 53% of men were smokers in 1985, but that this figure rose to 67% in 1993. Even 30% of women and 20% of boys aged 15 were smokers. This incidence is among the highest in the world, the European population average being 30%. Of all men aged 35, it is estimated that 20% will die of smoking-related diseases by the age of 69.
- In Europe as a whole, 2 million people are estimated to be heavy users of psychotic drugs. Young people are the main users, with increasing

cases of poisoning, suicide and premature death. Around 40% of drugs users have AIDS/HIV. This is expanding markedly in Belarus, the Russian Federation and Ukraine. The number of adolescent drug users increased ten-fold from the late 1980s to the late 1990s. They have a far greater rate of substance abuse than the general population. In Svetlogorsk, in Belarus, the grim industrial landscape is still contaminated by radioactive fallout from the Chernobyl nuclear disaster. It was founded in the 1960s as a model industrial centre. Some new migrants were from Central Asia, with traditional skills in growing opium poppies. Gypsy dealers now manufacture and sell it on the streets for very low sums. Used needles are found everywhere and drug dealers even push drugs in the hospital wards reserved for teenage addicts. Initially the police tried to arrest the suspected users and to test them forcibly for AIDS, but the problem spread quickly in spite of this. Western initiatives such as exchanging used needles and educating young people about drugs and the ways in which AIDS is spread have had limited success.

The World Health Organisation (WHO) has produced comprehensive reports on monitoring alcohol, drug and tobacco abuse and on their effects in 173 countries. It is a growing problem worldwide.

e) Debt and structural adjustment policies in LEDCs

Many LEDCs borrowed money for ambitious capital projects in the 1970s and 1980s, when international financial institutions, such as development banks, were happy to lend to them at low interest rates. With time, interest rates rose sharply while revenues from their main exports of commodities such as sugar, coffee or tin, for example, fell just as fast. The problem of 'servicing' this debt has, for many LEDCs, become a major part of their GNP outlay. It has now reached the stage where many LEDCs repay more in debts than they receive in aid. In some cases, even more borrowing has been necessary in order to discharge the debt.

But in order to secure a loan from the International Monetary Fund (IMF) the country must pledge itself to re-arrange its economic structure in order to concentrate on earning foreign currency through export earnings, rather than to spend money on social projects such as health and education. Public hospitals and health centres were sold to the private sector, which priced them out of the reach of poor people. This means that the vast majority of people in LEDCs, apart from the privileged elite, face the prospect of deteriorating healthcare, after a period of hope in the 1970s.

This arrangement with the IMF is known as an **Structural Adjustment Policy (SAP)**. The effects of this situation are felt all over the developing world:

- In Mozambique, the Maputo Central Hospital is rife with corruption (Hanlon 1999). Only by resorting to bribery could an X-ray be carried out. Nurses' wages are below the poverty line, and there is little equipment. In 1975 it was a showpiece, providing good quality healthcare for all. Unfortunately, the country became involved in a war with South Africa and had to borrow money to finance it. By 1991 the IMF ordered Mozambique to initiate an SAP, as it was so much in debt. This meant cutting back on basics like public sector pay. In 1992 the debt was $7 billion of which $350 million per year was meant to service the debt. The annual payments were less than that, with the balance being added to the total. This meant that the government was repaying $275,000 in debt services each day, but only $100,000 for the health service. Less than $20,000 went to the three biggest hospitals. Since then, the Jubilee 2000 group has been working hard to get debts cancelled so that investment in health can begin properly again.

- In Western Mexico, a local project had identified a major cause of infant mortality in peasant families as poor nutrition (Werner 2000). Half the crop had to be given to their landlord. Putting pressure on the landlord they secured better, irrigated land which enabled the IMR to fall from 340/1,000 to 60/1,000. Unfortunately, by the 1990s, Mexico's SAP needed to be serviced by an increases in cash crops. The farmers lost their land and migrated to slums in the cities.

f) Indigenous peoples

The problems of **indigenous peoples**, usually a tiny minority in a total population of former 'colonists', are particularly hard to resolve. Even though newcomers might have been in the area for several centuries, the impact they have had on the lives of those who have always lived a traditional **subsistence** life in the area in question continues to be adverse. Hunting, gathering and herding become increasingly impossible. With their way of life, so finely attuned to the local environment, fundamentally altered by wholesale environmental change (such as mining, urban and industrial development) there is little left for the indigenous peoples. Not only do physical illnesses result, but also mental problems. The frequent scarcity of healthcare for them does little to help, as the following shows:

- The history of the health of Native Americans and the Inuit in Canada, described by Rosenberg (2000) charts this decline. From the first contact these peoples had with Europeans in the sixteenth century, diseases such as measles and syphilis, to which they had no immunity, combined with new dietary influences, had devastating effects on morbidity and mortality rates. Enforced removal from traditional areas to 'reserves' which were often remote and marshy or polluted and the consequent lack of resources for their traditional way of life compounded an already grim state of affairs. The incidence of diabetes and heart disease became very much higher in these peoples as a result. Most of them live well below the low income cut-off line (LICO). What medical services do exist today are often poor and lacking in cultural sensitivity.

• The situation among the native peoples of Siberia, such as the Entsy who lived by trapping and herding not far from the Arctic Ocean, is graphically described by the local doctor to Thubron (2000):

'It's got desperate here. This used to be a fur-trading village, and was a reindeer collective in Khrushchev's day. But you see it now!' A coal-black pond glistened with discarded vodka bottles. 'The reindeer pastures have been ruined by acid rain . . .from the nickel-processing factories at Norilsk . . .People here are close to starving . . . .You'd think this place quiet, but it's the most troublesome in the world . . .these people fight . . .it's vodka of course. So there are ulcers and liver diseases.'

His hospital was a low wooden ark. It had no running water and its lavatory was a hole in the ground. It was almost without equipment . . .three part-time nurses tended the five children in its narrow iron beds . . . .More than half the population (of 500), mostly Entsy with a few Russians, was unemployed.

Summary

1. The epidemiological transition shows the changes in disease types in a country. These change from infectious diseases such as polio and measles to non-communicable diseases such as cancer, heart disease and, later, to degenerative diseases such as Alzheimer's.
2. This sequence is linked to progressive economic development, with MEDCs having arrived slowly at the final stages, but NICs having achieved the same results much more rapidly. LEDCs are still dominated by infectious diseases.
3. The epidemiological transition can explain variations in health and welfare up to a point, but the volume of health spending is another important variable.
4. Measurement of inequalities can make use of a variety of data. Deprivation indices can be valuable tools in planning health policy. Composite indices are a useful way of assessing global health status, but infant mortality rate (IMR) and under-five mortality rate (U5 IMR) are the most sensitive indicators of population health.
5. Richard Wilkinson maintains that increases in GNP do not result in a corresponding rise in life expectancy once the majority of the population has achieved a 'minimum material standard of living'. Thereafter, it is *equality* of provision that has most influence on the health of the entire population.
6. Patterns of life expectancy follow the general pattern of privileged core and disadvantaged periphery on a variety of scales.
7. The World Health Organisation (WHO) league table 2000 assesses the performance of 191 health systems in terms of overall population health, health inequalities, patient satisfaction and how different income groups are served.

8. Julian Tudor Hart's Inverse Care Law notes that the availability of good medical care varies in inverse proportion to the need for it. Territorial justice is the reverse situation. This was attempted in planned economies.

9. Doctors tend to prefer to live and practise in more favoured areas; it is hard to redress the balance.

10. The poor have little systematic healthcare and are less likely to seek help. Relative poverty means that they are unable to live in areas with good medical care, neither can they afford to pay, nor to be insured, in countries where free health cover is not available. In very poor societies it is often the provision of basic hygiene measures that are most effective in improving health. Traditional healers still play an important role, especially when trained in basic medical techniques.

11. Women are most vulnerable in poorer societies because childbirth and pregnancy are still very dangerous. Rather than the provision of more hospital units, UNICEF suggests that four simple interventions would make dramatic improvements to alarmingly high maternal and perinatal mortality rates.

12. Homelessness puts people at risk of many physical and mental illnesses. Frequent moves mean that continuity of care is difficult. Refugees experience every kind of hardship, with minimal assistance, if any.

13. Drug abuse is particularly acute in the CIS (former Soviet Union) where smoking, alcoholism and drug abuse have grown rapidly since 1990. Healthcare has become far less effective during this time.

14. Debt and Structural Adjustment Policies (SAPs) arranged to repay LEDC debts to MEDC institutions such as the International Monetary Fund (IMF) mean that a country concentrates spending on export-earning activities and 'servicing' its debt. This means that health and welfare budgets are slashed for the majority of the population.

15. Indigenous peoples still suffer greatly from 'colonial' invasions of many centuries ago. They lose their traditional land resources and their subsistence way of life is destroyed. Living on reserves in remote and often polluted areas, many are unemployed. Healthcare is patchy and inadequately tailored to their needs.

Suggested essay or report title

What factors influence access to healthcare?

The section on essay or report writing at the end of Chapter 2 contains a great deal of general information. Consult it, in addition to the specific details given here!

Choice of title

- It is good news and bad news:

  - The good news is that you have much more scope for planning an essay or report along the lines *you* want, as the title is general.
  - The bad news is that the title is so general that the examiners will

expect you to think of many different angles to the question. Putting these together can be a difficult job, as you have to be certain of your sequence of ideas.

- Consider the key words: *factors, access* and *healthcare* in relation to the generalisation. This will be a possible structure for you to follow.

- The theoretical background will relate to the epidemiological transition and its global pattern, to the Inverse Care Law and its opposite (territorial justice) and to geographical distance.

Research

- Make a copy of the relevant parts of the chart showing the chapter outline (Frontispiece I) on to A3 paper to give you a framework.
- List each source as you use it.
- Your case studies have to cover both *distance itself as a factor* in addition to all the *socio-economic factors* which make access even worse.
- The case studies must be from a range of LEDCs and NICs, MEDCs and former planned economies.
- The key words must have clear definitions.
- The possible links between theories and case studies should be drawn on the framework diagram.

Planning

See Chapter 2 for some general hints.

- The structure of your ideas must be clear. You could look at the ideal situation (territorial justice) by seeing how successful attempts to deliver it have been in planned (communist) economies (Cuba, China, Russian Federation).
- The Inverse Care Law could then be discussed with the bulk of your case studies illustrating all the different *factors controlling healthcare access* for the following groups:
- the poor – inability to buy medicines (for HIV/AIDS in South Africa) or insurance (USA)
- the homeless – difficulty of registering with a GP (UK)
- women – inferior to men in many (LEDC) societies (India)
- IDUs – prisoners (Russian federation)
- indigenous peoples – remoteness and cultural factors (Canada).
- Your conclusion must return to the idea of territorial justice. Is there any area where it is actually working? Why? What hope is there for other societies in the light of emergent diseases and an ageing society? (see Chapter 5).

The part played by geography in exploring the impacts of disease

4

1 How disease affects societies

An individual can experience a range of illnesses, from a sub-clinical state of infection, which is scarcely noticeable, to an **acute** infection, which might remain until immunity is gained, or to a long-term problem which might become a **chronic** or fairly permanent disability. All these states are those of **morbidity**. The final way in which disease can affect an individual is to cause death or **mortality**.

Societies are made up of many individuals who may be in varying states of morbidity. This can have profound economic and social effects if they form part of the working population but are unable to contribute through ill health. The finality of death removes an individual from the family, the community and the workforce, but the need for care in chronic debilitating illnesses has a more lasting effect on those remaining. They have to replace the work done by the individual when well and also provide support during the illness. In LEDCs, this **burden of disease** is considerable, especially in agricultural communities at subsistence level. The social, environmental and economic responses to the HIV/AIDS pandemic and to sleeping sickness illustrate this. Although there have been some effective global **eradication programmes** for some infectious diseases, others are **re-emerging** as resistant strains. More worryingly still, there are wholly new **emergent diseases**, which are threatening both MEDCs and LEDCs.

a) Three approaches

The **mortality approach** to examining the effects of disease on societies measures their effects through the deaths that they cause. Infectious diseases are still among the top ten global killers (Figure 3.2).

Using morbidity, one way of looking at the impact of disease is to consider **disease incidence**, which charts the number of new cases of a diseases in a year (Cliff et al 1998). Here diarrhoea in children under the age of five is the most prominent; it also *kills* 3 million a year.

A second and perhaps more useful way is by **disease prevalence** – the total number of people with a condition or the disability resulting from it.

b) How does this affect the global pattern?

In 1991, the WHO introduced the concept of the **Global Burden of Disease** (Murray 1991). This emphasised the inevitable changes in the pattern of worldwide diseases as the result of LEDCs moving through the **epidemiological transition**. Thus, non-communicable diseases such as depression and heart disease are 'fast replacing infectious diseases and malnutrition as the main causes of disability and premature death'.

The WHO predicts that 70% of deaths in LEDCs will be from non-communicable diseases by 2020. Injuries will overtake infections as a second major cause.

Mental illness has long been underrated. Although not responsible for many actual *deaths*, it is indeed responsible for a much-diminished quality of life for about 11% of those who are sick. Addiction to tobacco and alcohol is an increasingly important factor, with men in the CIS and Eastern Europe facing a 28% risk of death from alcohol-related illness between 15 and 60. By 2020 WHO estimates that tobacco will have killed more people than the current AIDS/HIV epidemic.

Looking at general morbidity and mortality statistics does not give a true picture of a country's health status. This is because:

- statistics are rarely complete and do not give a detailed breakdown of causes of death annually;
- information about those with non-fatal symptoms such as blindness or dementia is rarely available;
- epidemiologists may well exaggerate mortality figures if it means obtaining more resources with which to fight disease.

The importance of **disability** in addition to morbidity and mortality is emphasised by WHO. Those factors which are important in causing disability are very different from those which kill, and yet disability is perhaps more important in affecting the health of a whole population.

Psychiatric conditions are far more important than was originally thought. The main conditions are: depression; alcohol abuse; schizophrenia; obsessive-compulsive disorder.

Depression alone affected 10% of people who had chronic (long-standing) disability. The WHO uses the term the **YLDs (Years Lived with a Disability)** to describe conditions which disable, not kill, but alter the quality of life, often at its end. All mental illness accounted for 28% of all YLDs. This is most common in MEDCs and LEDCs, except for sub-Saharan Africa, possibly because of the low life expectancy here).

Alcohol abuse is the leading cause of male disability in MEDCs and fourth in LEDCs. The other conditions that were important as a cause of YLDs are: anaemia; falls; road traffic accidents; lung diseases; osteoarthritis.

There are important differences in **disease prevalence** as children approach adulthood. Women obviously suffer from childbearing, especially in LEDCs. Worldwide, reproductive health problems cause

30% of YLDs in all women aged 15–44. In LEDCs, 50% of premature deaths in this age group are related to this cause, including unsafe abortion and chlamydia. Most of this represents the loss of otherwise healthy women, which has a profound impact on the society and economy. Nonetheless, the leading **disease burden** for women is caused by depression in both MEDCs and LEDCs; this is followed by suicide in the LEDCs. The priorities must be, therefore, to target women's psychological health.

Road traffic accidents are the biggest cause of deaths and disability worldwide for men. They will soon kill more people across the world than HIV/AIDS, cancer, conflict or famine (Peek 2001). Around 800,000 people are killed on roads every year; at least 23 million are injured. Of these totals, 85% are often bus passengers from LEDCs. Depression is the second killer, followed by alcohol abuse, violence, TB and war.

By 2020, **mental health** will account for 15% of the disease burden, tobacco 9% and heart disease 6% (the leading projected disease). The WHO comments: 'This is a global health emergency that many governments have yet to confront.'

A report from the Global Forum for Health Research (BMJ 2000) claims that less than 10% of the world's health research budget is spent on conditions which actually account for 90% of the world's burden of disease. The forum called for this total of $56 billion to be spent more equitably.

The forum's chairman, Professor Adetokunbo Lucas, commented:

> the world's two biggest killer diseases – pneumonia and diarrhoeal disease – illustrate the extreme mis-match between the disease burden and the funding of research and development. Although these two killers represent about 11% of the total global burden of disease, only about a fifth of 1% of health research funding is spent on them.

Individual countries need to take a wider view as travel, **emergent diseases and resistant microbes** become important. Multiple agencies to generate new funding, for example the Medicines for Malaria Venture producing new anti-malarial drugs, are the way forward. The Bill Gates Foundation has pledged to spend several million dollars over five years. The World Bank and many MEDC governments support the Global Forum itself. Spending on defence is contrasted by the WHO with spending need for disease control in Figure 4.1.

c) The size of the infectious disease burden in the USA

Cliff et al (1998) have estimated the size of the infectious disease burden in the USA in the mid-1980s. The Centers for Disease Control and Prevention (CDC) estimate that 83% of all deaths are indirectly

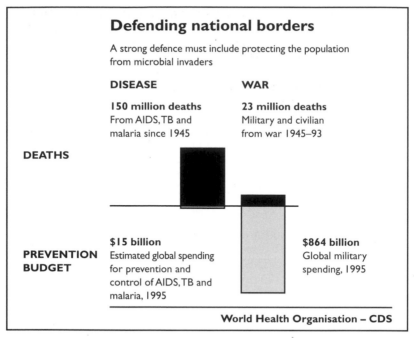

Figure 4.1 **Spending on defence and spending need for disease control –
WHO**
(Source: BMJ 2000 320; 1228)

caused by infection, in that they contribute to mortality from degenerative disease; this clouded the picture. Subsequent research concluded that there were 740 million infections a year in the USA, which
caused 200,000 deaths. 'Such infections resulted in more than $17 bil-
lion annually in direct costs, not including costs of deaths, lost wages
and other indirect costs.'

Plans to prevent up to 150,000 deaths a year from infection are
under way. The largest number of deaths (50,000) was caused by
pneumonia and similar infections. The top infection for morbidity
was the common cold, caused by the rhinovirus (125 million);
influenza had 20 million cases.

2 The AIDS pandemic

I was standing at the end of a squalid bed in the Mam Yemo
Hospital, Kinshasa, Zaire, watching a woman die. She could only
be about twenty-five I guessed. Her practically motionless form
was stretched out on a stained mattress. There were no sheets to
cover her nakedness. I swatted at the flies, which buzzed relent-
lessly round my ears. She had lost her hair; her face was sallow,

and her eyes sunken. Her lips were studded with raw sores. Her tongue must have caused her great pain: when I examined it more closely, I could see that it was encrusted with the yeast infection we now know to be so common in people afflicted with terminal AIDS. Her skin was stretched tautly over her bones like an unpainted canvas over a frame. In places it was sown with the livid, bulging blotches of Kaposi's sarcoma, a cancer of the blood vessels in the skin, widely seen in AIDS patients. Over other parts of her body, bedsores had excavated extensive suppurating craters.

As accustomed as I was to seeing the terminally sick, the plight of this young woman overwhelmed me. She epitomised for me the emergence in Africa of the discordant modern world where none of the old rules applied.

Joseph McCormick and Susan Fisher-Hoch, *The Virus Hunters*,
1997

AIDS is indubitably the plague of the late 20th century.

Meade and Earikson 2000

a) What is AIDS?

HIV is the **human immunodeficiency virus** and AIDS is the **acquired immunodeficiency syndrome** which it causes. HIV is a slow **retrovirus**, which means that not only does it take years to show symptoms but it also invades the white cells by literally 'writing' the structure of itself *backwards* (*retro*) into them and reproducing itself *inside* them instead. These cells normally produce antibodies and are the body's main defence against disease. Without them the body becomes the target of everyday infections and cell changes which cause cancer; it is suffering from AIDS.

b) Where did it come from?

The virus evolved in sub-Saharan Africa, crossing over from a subgroup of chimpanzees to people somewhere in Central Africa possibly in the 1930s. This could have been from contaminated meat or a bite from a pet. Another suggestion is that that the virus had long been present in the human population in Central Africa but on a localised scale until the twentieth century. A combination of international travel, urbanisation, contaminated blood and intravenous drug use (IDU) produced a growing **pandemic**.

c) How does AIDS spread?

Today there are eight sub-types (or clades) of the virus. One of them (B1) is the only form present in North America, Latin America,

Europe, Japan and Australia. This indicates that there was a single source, which spread in the 1970s. In Africa, E is the most prevalent clade. It is the most transmissible, which explains why AIDS in Africa is so devastating. Vaccination against HIV is virtually impossible; not only are there so many clades, but each also mutates (changes its form) very frequently.

The virus spreads through exchange of body fluids:

* through unprotected sex – homosexual or bisexual men or prostitutes of either sex can have a higher risk as they have more partners;
* through use of contaminated needles by IDU;
* through the transfusion of contaminated blood (important for haemophiliacs, who need regular blood transfusions as their blood lacks a clotting agent);
* from mother to child either in the womb or by breast feeding.

The disease seems to start in small high-risk groups, such as gay men, IDUs or prostitutes. It will spread within the group by **assortive mating** but **disassociative mating** (outside the group) will cause it to move into society as a whole.

d) How can geography explain its spread?

Mapping the disease in its early stages in the 1980s in the USA was difficult as the issue of patient confidentiality prevented data from being released (Meade & Earikson 2000).

The pattern of spread from large cities into the surrounding states and thence to rural areas in all major continents is one of **hierarchical diffusion** with a linear element along interstate highways. In analysing these trends, geographers can predict the next stage and therefore assist with effective resource planning. If a group of people are distant from the source of infection, they can enhance the protective effect of the distance by taking extra precautions. One of the most successful is that of using peer educators, in the form of commercial sex workers.

e) Where does it occur?

In the early stages, AIDS was regarded as a 'Gay Plague' or confined mainly to IDUs by many in the MEDCs, which prevented the heterosexual or 'straight' community from regarding it seriously. Education about 'safe sex' was disregarded. In LEDCs, mainly in Africa, heterosexual transfer was common; drugs were not. Many in the West disregarded these facts. As it did not at first appear in Asia, many there thought they had a racial immunity. Even when Thailand was hit, there was little publicity because of fears from the tourism industry.

In 2000, record year for cases, 5.2 million people were infected with HIV and 2.8 million died of AIDS. Of the total number living with HIV (36.6 million), 23.3 million live in sub-Saharan Africa (*The Week* 2000). More than 40% of the HIV infection today is in poor women. In many US cities, AIDS is the leading cause of death in women aged 15–44.

The highest rates in Asia are in Thailand, Burma (now Myanmar) and Cambodia. East Asia and Oceania have a fairly low incidence. Brazil and Mexico have the bulk of cases in Latin America. The infection has not been long in the Middle East and North Africa; infection rates are low. The disease is spreading in a horrifying way in the Russian Federation and in Eastern Europe as a whole. There are many infected in Western Europe; these are mainly male. In the United States and Canada 20% of HIV infection is now female.

f) Is there a pattern to HIV/AIDS?

There seem to be two main patterns in the world:

1. **Type 1**, associated with MEDCs, involving transmission by homosexuals, IDUs, contaminated blood, and women infected by their partners and their babies. As these groups can be clearly identified there is no general epidemic threat.
2. **Type 2**, associated with LEDCs, especially African countries, involving heterosexual transmission, especially through prostitutes, contaminated blood, and rituals such as circumcision. Drugs are usually absent.

Those in lower socio-economic groups are those who suffer most in either pattern.

g) Is there any hope of a cure?

At present the hope of a **vaccine** is distant (by 2010?). However, there is research to show that a group of Kenyan prostitutes seemed to have particularly strong white (T cell) responses to the virus. Their possible 'immunity' is being studied. The other strategy is **drug therapy**. AZT, the so-called 'triple therapy', costs around $10,000 a year for each sufferer. Even nevirapine, a slightly cheaper drug, is beyond the means of many poorer countries. While these are not cures and have severe side effects, they do represent a way of prolonging life for many in the MEDCs.

For those in poorer societies in LEDCs and FPEs, there is little prospect of therapy, even with drug companies reducing the costs, as happened in the test case against 39 international drugs companies in South Africa in April 2001. Here the best plan is AIDS awareness education, which has been very successful in some areas. A great deal depends on political will. Those countries with a positive attitude, seeking the help of NGOs and international funding, have made impressive progress. Those countries where the government is in flat denial of the problem have experienced great pain and suffering already. Such is the slow nature of the virus that for many, regrettably, the worst is yet to come, whatever is done in the short term.

CASE STUDIES

Figure 4.2 shows the factors affecting HIV/AIDS in:

- **New Zealand**, an MEDC remote from the main infected areas, which is well-resourced to deal with its small number of cases;
- **The Russian Federation**, a former planned economy (FPE) from the old Soviet Union where IDUs and prostitution have produced the highest rate of HIV infection in the world in the last decade;
- **Thailand**, an LEDC where careful strategies targeting vulnerable groups have been successful in the face of a high infection rate;
- **Myanmar (formerly Burma)**, an LEDC with a repressive military regime, which has suppressed democracy and freedom of information. Refusal to allow sex education or to spend adequately on HIV/AIDS awareness and prevention has led to untold suffering. It has been described as:

the epicentre of the AIDS epidemic in Asia

John Dwyer of the AIDS society in Asia

characterised by a political culture marked by state violence and corruption, chronic civil war and insurgency, and an explosive and recent AIDS epidemic...the junta (military regime) shows no sign of progress, but the HIV epidemic will not wait.

Chris Beyrer 1999

- **South Africa**, an African LEDC with the time bomb of AIDS expected in the next decade as the result of governmental incompetence and denial:

for many years, thousands of South Africans, who might have lived long and productive lives, will be dying because of the irresponsible policies of a culpably misguided government.

The Economist 2001

Figure 4.2 The progress of HIV/AIDS in five selected countries

I. Main groups affected; **2.** Rates of infection and mortality. Future
projections; **3.** Methods of spread; **4.** Main centres and diffusion patterns;
5. Government attitudes; **6.** Treatment and/or prevention. Types of funding

New Zealand (date of first infection early 1980s)
I. mainly aged 25–45; asylum seekers; male homosexuals; 3 HIV+ babies;
prisoners; IDUs
2. 1999 – 23 cases; 1999 – 1,200 adults and 532 AIDS–related deaths; rates
now levelling off
3. MSM (homosexual contact); plans needed for heterosexual diffusion; IDUs in
prison (need condoms, methadone – heroine substitute – and needles; general
condom use low (20%)
4. from cities to rural areas
5. changed from helping chronic sick to dealing with housing and jobs for
those HIV+ victims with long-term therapy; Dept of Correction must provide
help for prisoners
6. long-term (triple therapy) – must be careful to avoid drug resistance

Russian Federation (date of first infection 1990)
I. IDUs (3–4 million prisoners); prostitutes; gay and bisexual men
2. highest rate in world; 2,000–3,000 infected per month; 70,000 registered
with HIV+; 4,000,000 estimated as undiagnosed
3. casual sex in gay clubs; IDUs (especially in prison); prostitution
4. in Baltic ports (e.g. Kalingrad) – easy to get heroin; widespread STDs
(sexually transmitted diseases) show how HIV could spread too
5. AIDS victims 'should be punished'; Soviet government ignored problems;
Orthodox church objected to safe sex TV programme; Ministry of Health now
recognizes epidemic; inadequate strategies until recently; conservative
attitude forbade sex education in schools
6. too poor to pay for drug therapy – $1.6 million available for 2000 (1/1000
of US spending on AIDS); must target whole population to prevent
heterosexual spread; ignorance of transmission methods – must have
education; charity projects include 'Body Positive' funding for TV campaign,
We and You campaign; $20 million needed by 2003 – funded by UN AIDS
programme ($750,000 in 2000) and World Bank loan ($150,000)

Thailand (date of first infection 1984)
I. commercial sex workers (CSWs)/prostitutes – low condom use; IDUs;
economically active (wage earners and tax payers) costing $11 billion in
2000 (representing care of orphans and care from spouses and lost work);
many infected workers coming home to Thailand to die; grandparents of
orphans (often poor and landless and retired) looking after them
2. 1993 – 30% CSW population had AIDS; 1999 – 950,000 were HIV+ and 66,000
died of AIDS
3. mainly from CSWs to rest of population
4. from returning migrants on northern border; from main cities
5. awareness campaign; 1991 – 100% condom programme to supply 60 million
condoms free; AIDS awareness to conquer threat to tourist industry
6. PWH (people with HIV groups); Buddhist monks provide support; rates of
condom use: 1991 – 36% men with CSWs/2001 – 90% men with CSWs; UN and Red
Cross and other NGOs help to break culture of silence; income-generating
projects for grandparents of orphans: chickens/crafts to help with schooling
costs

Myanmar (Burma) (date of first infection 1988)

1. women from ethnic minority groups returning from enforced work in Thailand as CSWs; IDUs (illegal to possess syringes so use 'tea stalls' for sharing needles (Myanmar is one of the world's largest heroin exporters); prostitutes (illegal – attracting 10-year jail sentence and 100,000 convictions per year – but flourishing); prisoners (see above) – 96% are HIV+ and share needles; blood transfusions in rural areas unsafe; prostitution spreading in jade and ruby mines in North: young men migrate there for work in dry season, become UDUs and infect wives on return

2. 1995 – 1% population HIV+ (400,000); 2000 government estimate – 66,463 HIV+ and UN estimate – 800,000; IMR (infant mortality rate) now 81/1,000 (Thailand 31/1,000)

3. CSWs; IDUs; prisoners; blood transfusion; migrant workers

4. from the northern border to India, China, Thailand (and drugs); from jade and ruby mines

5. no democracy since 1988 – military junta; 1990 Aung San Suu Kyi and NLD (National League for Democracy) wins election but has been under house arrest for many years subsequently as SLORC junta (now National Peace and Defence Committee) are still in power; total censorship of media – claims to have control for health and education: minister Major General Ket Sein said 'the best way to control AIDS is to control yourself, as there is no medicine to cure the disease'; tolerates laundering of drugs revenues; SLORC involved in selling poor women as CSWs; many health professionals murdered by SLORC; US sanctions since 1997 limit medicine supply; government spends 60% of revenue on defence

South Africa (date of first infection 1987)

1. rape victims) only 1/35 rapes are reported); migrant workers to goldmines; migrants' wives (on their return); CSWs; children – many with congenital HIV+ status and orphaned – roam around in gangs with no hope for the future; the malnourished – more easily infected

2. 4 million HIV + and 2 million children (congenital) by 2010; 2005 – 365,000 deaths from AIDS forecast; 2010 – 600,000 deaths forecast; 8 million infected by 2005; life expectancy is 60 (2001) and will be 40 (2008)

3. diagnosis is inexpert – can be confused with malaria/TB/cholera; workers migrate to goldmines, sleep with CSWs and return to wives; men and women have many sexual partners; no treatment to prevent MTC (mother to child transmission) available for pregnant women

4. migrant workers from goldmine townships back to homelands

5. 1999 – in denial; Mandela government too embarrassed; Mbeki government took up several theories: of Peter Duesberg and Geshekler that only malnutrition was to blame, that it was a CIA conspiracy, that drugs companies wanted to profit too highly from treatment; subsequent policy blunders: advancing cheap 'miracle cures' (virodene) – refusing to make AZT available for pregnant women, refusal to allow use of nevirapine until September 2000, rejection of discounted drugs, doctors forbidden to treat HIV+ children; lack of condoms; now medical insurance companies must accept all applicants

6. palliative care (no remedial treatment) e.g. children's hospice in Johannesburg – only 18 beds/one death a week/400% turnover; AIDS-related illnesses will cost the economy from 28 billion rand (2001) to 38 billion rand (2010); private sector bill up by 25% (20% S. Africans have private medicine); economic growth will be down by 0.4% per year ($22 billion less by 2010); goldmines will lose 3% of workforce; other companies may lose 3% of workforce (and death benefits and disability pensions)

3 Sleeping sickness

a) What is sleeping sickness?

The disease is caused by a **trypanosome**, a single-cell parasite transmitted by the **tsetse fly**. There are two forms of the disease found in humans: West African sleeping sickness (*t. brucei gambiense*) and East African sleeping sickness (*t. brucei rhodesiensi*) and one in domestic animals such as cattle, horses and goats (*t. brucei*). There is a man–fly–man transmission cycle, but sometimes pigs, antelopes and game are secondary reservoirs (Netdoctor 2000, CDC Factsheets 1999 and 2000).

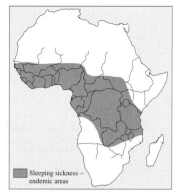

Sleeping sickness – endemic areas

Figure 4.3 **Endemic sleeping sickness areas**
(Source: www.fit-for-travel.de)

b) What geographical factors influence its occurrence?

It is a disease of tropical Africa. The map (Figure 4.3) shows the main areas affected. The WHO estimates that some 36 countries are at risk. Different species of the tsetse fly favour different types of environment; some prefer scrub, while others favour forests near lakes and rivers or deep tropical forest. The disease is thought to have been endemic for thousands of years, but it was only when the basin of the Congo river was opened up by European colonial powers in the nineteenth century, with trading posts established along its banks, that it began to spread. Migration by pastoral nomads also became confined by new colonial boundaries (Africa Unification Front, World Socialist Website 1998).

In the 1960s, it was all but eradicated by screening the population, trapping flies and the use of pesticides. This tempted farmers to move their crops and animals into formerly infested areas. All this changed when civil war and unrest came to many of the countries where the disease was endemic, following independence. Formal controls and the funding to carry them out were abandoned. Now the disease is spreading exponentially, with 25,000 new cases each year and 60 million people thought to be at risk. Most of these are in Highly

Indebted Poor Countries (HIPCs), which are crippled by international debt (FAO 1996).

In the Democratic Republic of the Congo 20,000 cases were reported in 1995, but the WHO estimate was more like 250,000. This is more devastating than mortality from AIDS. In Angola the reported incidence was 2,478 in 1995 but the WHO estimate was 100,000 (Angola Peace Monitor 2000). In the Sudan there were 12,000 cases in one county; in some villages 45% of the population was infected. The figure was 4% in 1988, ten years earlier (Medecins Sans Frontières 1999).

c) What are the symptoms?

Once bitten by the tsetse fly, the victim experiences a sore (chancre) around the site of the bite within a fortnight. Fever and swollen lymph nodes follow this. The disease progresses slowly; within a few months the parasite makes its way into the central nervous system. The results are sleep disturbance, confusion and a profound personality change. Without treatment, death is usually inevitable within a year.

d) What are the social effects of the disease?

Since the disease is fatal, it is possible that large areas of central Africa could be completely depopulated. It is the chief cause of mortality in many areas. Once they have contracted the disease, and especially in its latter stages, victims are unable to work and need care from their families, even if they are receiving treatment in hospital. In some areas, whole villages lie deserted, as people have fled, abandoning their livestock and crops. Women tend to suffer more than men, since they must rely on their husbands for care. If they seek treatment from traditional healers they may have ritual cuts on their faces, which leave deep scars. This and the stigma attached to the disease means that even if they do recover, their chances of marriage are slight. Children's school performance is badly affected; they often have severe behavioural disturbance.

e) What are its economic effects?

The WHO estimate that the burden of the disease in terms of lost working years is 1.47 million. It is thus a major obstacle to development. Without draft animals it has been impossible to intensify agriculture in many parts of central Africa. An estimated 10 million square kilometres of the country with fertile soil and sufficient rainfall cannot be farmed because of the disease. Loss of livestock from the parasite is put at $5,000 million a year. Looking after sick relatives removes yet more people from the agricultural workforce. By the premature death of a family member, the average rural inhabitant loses 10 years of income (around $1,615).

f) Is there the hope of a cure?

The cause of sleeping sickness was established in 1901. In the 1920s a French epidemiologist realised that whole communities had to be treated, rather than individuals. What is needed is to sterilise the human reservoir and to destroy the vector (the tsetse fly). With pyramid-shaped traps baited with pyrethrum insecticide it was possible to reduce levels of the disease in the Masai's grazing grounds in Kenya such that their goats' milk yield improved. With around 7,000 years of infection there must be some resistance too amongst the wild game. Biological control is a potential option.

For humans the treatment is as follows:

1. **Drug therapy with melarsoprol**: this costs around $150 per course, takes 26 days to administer and, since it contains arsenic, has horrific side effects which are dangerous and painful. The entire treatment regime takes two years. Around 30% of the cases in Uganda are now resistant to it.
2. **Drug therapy with eflornithine**: this costs $300 per course and can be effective in the later stages.

The WHO estimates that it costs $1,000 per person for treatment. A total of $30 million is necessary to fight the disease. Only $1 million has been forthcoming so far. The countries involved are crippled by debt and conflict, in any case. Political stability is their first requirement, and the simple tests and affordable drugs, which might put an end to this disease, are not yet on the horizon (E.T. online).

4 Global eradication?

a) How can a transmission model help in the eradication of infectious diseases?

Eradication refers to the total removal of a disease from the planet. A number of control strategies exist for infectious diseases (Cliff, Haggett & Smallman-Raynor 1998). A measles epidemic follows the Hamer–Soper model discussed in Chapter 2. Those at risk have their numbers increased by new births. People who have not had the disease (suceptibles) mix with those who have it (infectives). Infectives then get better (recovereds) or die. The epidemic maintains itself when there is a sufficient mixing rate of susceptibles with infectives.

Protection against infection spread can take two forms (Figure 4.4). 'Geographical' methods interrupt mixing by imposing a protective spatial barrier: restriction or quarantine (B and C).

The second form provides some immunity from the disease (thereby short-circuiting the route from 'infected' to 'recovered' status) by mass immunisation or vaccination such as for polio or measles, which will be described later in this chapter (A and D).

b) What is the relationship between endemic infectious diseases and population size?

As was shown in Chapter 2, there has to be a sufficient reservoir of 'infecteds' in a population in order for a disease to remain **endemic**. In sparsely populated areas, **epidemics** will occur only by the immigration of new 'infecteds'.

c) What spatial strategies are there for controlling infectious disease?

The global eradication of **smallpox**, as described later, used the technique of **progressive reduction** of the areas in which it occurred. The diagram (Figure 4.4) shows four stages by which this can be achieved:

- local elimination breaks the disease chain by vaccination (A)
- defensive isolation builds a spatial barrier around a disease-free area (B)
- offensive containment is the reverse of the above, as it aims to halt the localised spread of a disease into a larger area, using vaccination and isolation (C).

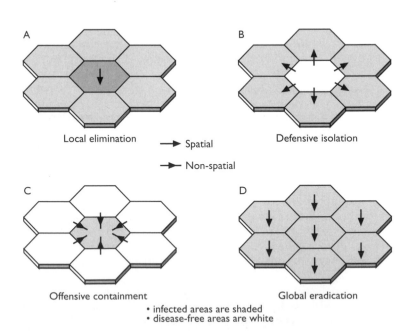

Local elimination   ➡ Spatial   Defensive isolation

➡ Non-spatial

Offensive containment   Global eradication

- infected areas are shaded
- disease-free areas are white

Figure 4.4 **Protection against infection spread**
(Source: *Deciphering Global Epidemics*, Cliff, A., Haggett, P. and Smallman-Raynor, M. C.U.P. 2000)

- global eradication occurs from combining the three methods described; by reducing the size of infected areas, and increasing those which are disease-free (D).

According to Cliff, Haggett & Smallman-Raynor (1998), 'Total extinction of a bacillus or virus from the planet rests on a global control programme'. This must reduce the sizes of the populations at risk to levels below those at which the chain of infection can operate.

d) Can there be spatial forecasts of disease spread?

Using **probability modelling**, Gould (1995) – quoted by Cliff et al 1996 – attempted to predict the future pattern of AIDS in the USA. He took as his starting point the distribution of AIDS in the 102 largest cities in the country and superimposed the pattern of internal air travel on to this. In this way he could 'model' the contacts between places. The five largest cities 'exchanged' 13 million people between them in 1992. Predicting the probability of future exchanges was based on the observed pattern of AIDS in 1986.

A comparison of the prediction and the actual pattern is shown in Figure 4.5. Where the model over-predicted, there are older industrial towns with a high number of blue-collar workers with Catholic backgrounds. By contrast, the southern cities with high tourist populations were under-predicted. This technique will be

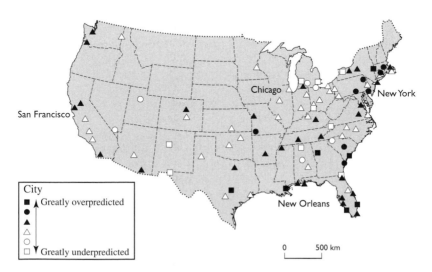

Figure 4.5 **Comparison of predicted and actual HIV/AIDS cases in the USA – white symbols (overpredicted); black symbols (underpredicted)**
(Source: Gould in Cliff, A., et al (ibid) 2000)

increasingly useful for constructing 'global early warning systems for the transmission of communicable disease', according to Cliff et al (1998).

e) Global eradication programmes

Smallpox

> Smallpox is ushered in with severe symptoms, a shivering fit, great depression of spirits and debility, languor, sickness, headache, pains in the back and loins and occasional delirium. After the above symptoms have lasted about three days the eruption shows itself, usually, mostly on the face and forehead, and wrists, unlike chickenpox ...on the appearance of the eruptional the above symptoms are aggravated and the danger begins ...the 'breaking out' is composed entirely of pustules containing matter ...more on the face than on any other part of the body ...there is generally a peculiar smell – an odour once smelt never to be forgotten...smallpox is highly contagious ... more than half the children under five years of age unprotected by vaccination die if they get smallpox.
>
> G.T. Wrench, *Chavasse's Advice to a Mother*, London, 1924

The 'death' of smallpox occurred in October 1977. This was the date of the last natural case (Fenner et al 1988 – quoted by Cliff et al 1998). This successful eradication of what for centuries had been a killer disease could be the possible blueprint for other eradication programmes.

The **eradication** of smallpox began in the 1960s. Before this, the main method of control had been by **mass vaccination**. Indeed, the very word 'vaccination' is derived from Edward Jenner's eighteenth-century experiments in inoculation. He used cowpox (Latin *vacca*: cow) material to induce an immunity to smallpox after noticing that milkmaids rarely contracted smallpox. Vaccination breaks the chain between infecteds and susceptibles, but this was the case only in MEDCs. LEDCs were still a potent reservoir. Even with the vaccination of 500 million people in India in the early 1960s, the disease continued to be endemic. This was owing to the reservoir of 10% of the population who had escaped vaccination, many of whom were under 15.

Consequently, a ten-year programme to eradicate smallpox was begun in 1967:

* the first step was mass vaccination
* the subsequent four-phase programme was preparatory, attack, consolidation and maintenance.

The maps in Figure 4.6 show how successful the programme was. The

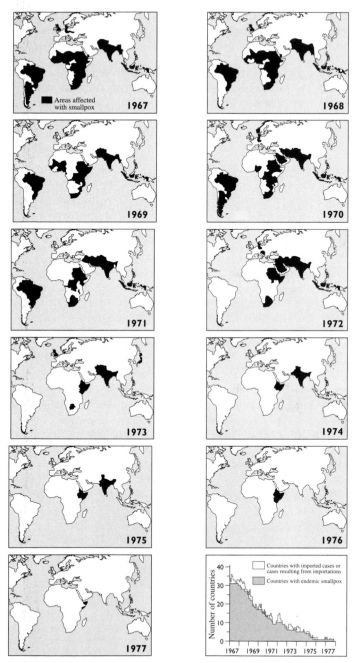

Figure 4.6 **Global eradication of smallpox under the WHO Intensified Programme 1967–77**
(Source: Fenner et al in Cliff et al (ibid) 2000)

last case was a man in Somalia in 1977 (Figure 4.7). Two years later the WHO announced that the world was clear of smallpox.

Polio

Poliomyelitis, or infantile paralysis, is caused by a number of viruses, which damage the motor nerves running from the spinal cord to the muscles. It was common in MEDCs until the mass immunisation in the late 1950s and early 1960s. In severe cases, victims had to be placed in an 'iron lung' for the rest of their lives, as even the respiratory muscles failed. In about 50% of cases there was permanent paralysis of the legs.

At the World Health Assembly in Geneva in 1988, WHO committed itself to ridding the world of polio (Figure 4.8). There were fewer than 2,000 reported cases in 2000, compared with 350,000 in 1988 (Figure 4.9), but WHO has pointed out that less than 15% of cases are actually reported. The plan is to eradicate polio by 2005 (Brundtland 2000) by:

1. intensifying immunisation
2. increasing surveillance to detect all cases
3. containing laboratory specimens safely
4. agreeing a timetable for national immunisation days
5. making routine immunisations where the wild virus may still persist.

This will be carried out by 10 million volunteers, joining forces with the Red Cross and the Red Crescent. Access must be made to all chil-

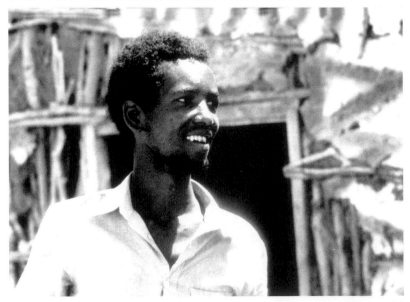

Figure 4.7 **The world's last naturally occuring smallpox case, a 23-year-old Somalian**

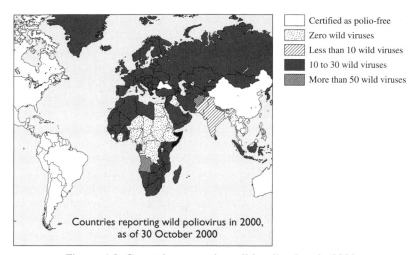

Figure 4.8 **Countries reporting wild polio virus in 2000**
(Source: Global Polio Initiative www.polioeradication.org)

dren and a further $450 million dollars of funding is needed. Each vaccine dose costs two cents, but more than 2 billion vaccines are required. There are great economic benefits to eradication for all countries. By the year 2015, $3 billion will be saved annually if there are no more cases left to treat.

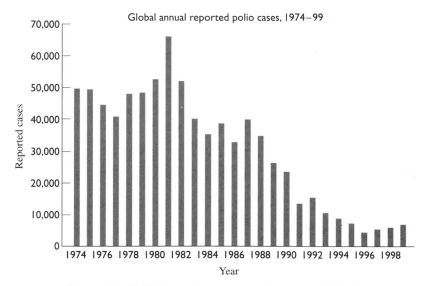

Figure 4.9 **Global annual reported polio cases, 1974–99**
(Source: WHO www.who.int/vaccines-surveillance/graphics)

Measles

Measles commences with the symptoms of the common cold ... these symptoms usually last three days before the eruption appears . . . .This consists of crescent-shaped areas of a dusky red hue; they usually appear first about the face and neck, then on the body and on the arms, and, lastly on the legs, and they are slightly raised above the surface of the skin . . . .They are formed by a peculiar grouping of several raised spots . . .often the spots run together and form large and quite irregular patches . . . .The face is swollen, more especially the eyelids, which are sometimes for a few days closed. The throat is red sore and swollen. The mucous or lining membrane of the bronchial tubes is always more or less inflamed, and the lungs themselves are sometimes infected. Ulcers may form on the eyes, or there may be inflammation around the eyeballs; abscesses are liable to form in the ears . . .and by spreading inwards may lead to inflammation of the brain. In fact the whole constitution is impaired and less resistant after an attack of measles.

G.T. Wrench, *Chavasse's Advice to a Mother,* London, 1924

Measles provides a very good example of the complex relationship between mortality, morbidity and major clinical interventions through vaccination, which, for measles became available after 1963.

A. Cliff, P. Haggett, and M. Smallman-Raynor, *Deciphering Global Epidemics*, CUP, Cambridge 1998

In 1990, the number of deaths from measles in MEDCs was 63. The **mortality rate** among children in these countries is generally 1 per 1,000. In 1990, WHO estimated that over 1.5 million deaths in LEDCs had been caused by measles (Cliff et al 1998). Here the mortality rate can be as high as 200 per 1,000, because of subsequent complications. In the USA attempts at **elimination** (stamping it out nationally) had been made in the 1960s. The programme went well until funds were switched to rubella (German measles) immunisation. Thereafter, the susceptibles in the population increased and so did the number of cases. Another attempt was made in the 1970s, but with constant additions to the population by immigration, elimination is not possible just yet. This is also due to the fact that the vaccine itself is only 80% effective.

In the UK a programme of 'triple vaccination' (MMR) was introduced in 1988 (Charter 2001). This offers protection against measles, mumps and rubella. The last is not serious in itself, but is likely to cause profound foetal abnormality if contracted in the first few weeks of pregnancy. Nine million children have had the vaccine but immunisation levels had fallen below 75% in some areas, making the possibility of an endemic reservoir likely.

The reason for the falling take-up of the MMR vaccine in the UK originated in the health scare over MMR in the USA in 1998. Claims that it caused brain damage were followed later by others, which linked it with the development of autism, a learning disability, and Crohn's disease, a chronic condition affecting the bowels. A large study undertaken in Finland over 18 years seemed to rule out any connections, but confidence is still weak in some quarters. Campaigners link it to 1,800 cases of autism.

The picture of measles vaccination is thus not as complete as that of polio (Figure 4.10)

5 Emerging and re-emergent diseases

Instead of disappearing at the end of the [epidemiological] transition, we find diseases once almost eradicated now opening new hospital wards. The most notorious of these is the multiple-drug-resistant new tuberculosis; but strains of MRSA (methicillin-resistant staphylococcus aureus) in hospitals threaten again to make them places to get sick. Children again die of intestinal fauna acquired in the meat and water of the most developed places.

Melinda Meade and Robert Earickson, *Medical Geography*, 2000

a) What are emerging and re-emerging diseases?

There are many factors which lie behind the rise in newly discovered or **emerging infectious diseases**. These also influence **re-emerging**

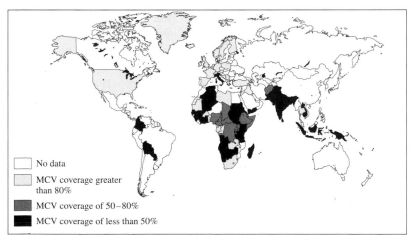

No data

MCV coverage greater than 80%

MCV coverage of 50–80%

MCV coverage of less than 50%

Figure 4.10 **Global immunisation coverage with measles-containing vaccine, based on WHO regional reports, 1998**
(Source: WHO www.who.int/vaccines-surveillance/graphics)

diseases (new, more resistant forms of infectious diseases which have been known for centuries). Ampel (quoted in Cliff et al 1998) suggests the main factors:

* the infections were present all along but were unrecorded as they were unrecognised: this may well be the case for Ebola virus (see later) or HIV/AIDS;
* the pathogens (disease agents) have always existed but are now more virulent (infectious) possibly due to mutation: the influenza pandemic at the end of the First World War was a vicious strain, killing more than the war itself did;
* changes in the environment and in human behaviour have created new situations in which diseases can flourish: toxic shock syndrome caused by failing to change tampons (sanitary protection) regularly;
* new epidemics arise when an infection arrives in a non-immune population: measles can wipe out remote indigenous peoples when they make contact with settlers, in Amazonia, for instance.

The table (Figure 4.11) shows the main developments over the last 20 years.

b) Can geography help to explain the rise of these diseases?

Some of the reasons why infectious disease has become more widespread are directly connected to medical practice, more especially to the use of medicinal drugs.

> If we fail to make wide and wise use of the medicines we have today, they will slip through our grasp due to anti-microbial resistance. It is the most telling sign that we have failed to take the threat of infectious diseases seriously …by over-using diseases-fighting drugs in developed nations and …by both misusing and under-using them in developing nations.
>
> David Heymann, *WHO*, June 2000

There are also issues which are directly related to land use change or to global warming which are highly significant geographically (Meade & Earickson 2000): deforestation; irrigation; dam building; agricultural intensification; road building; urbanisation; globalisation; pollution; industrialisation of food production.

c) Tuberculosis (TB) re-emerges

A global emergency?
The WHO declared TB to be a global emergency in 1993. The estimates in 1998 suggested that:

Re-emerging infections during the last two decades and factors contributing to their re-emergence

Disease or Agent	Factors in re-emergence
Viral	
Rabies	Breakdown in public health measures; changes in land use: travel
Bola/Dengue/dengue hemorrhagic fever	Transport, travel and migration; urbanisation
Yellow Fever	Drug and insecticide resistance; civil strife; lack of economic resources
Parasitic	
Schistosomiasis (bilharzia)	Dam construction, improved irrigation, and ecological changes favouring the snail host
Neurocysticercosis	Immigration
Acanthamebiasis	Introduction of soft contact lenses
Visceral leishmaniasis	War, population displacement, immigration, habitat changes favourable to the insect vector, an increase in immunocompromised human hosts
Malaria	Favourable conditions for mosquito vector
Toxoplasmosis	Increase in immunocompromised human hosts
Giardiasis	Increased use of child-care facilities
Echinococcosis	Ecological changes that affect the habitats of the intermediate (animal) hosts
Bacterial	
Group A Streptococcus	Uncertain
Trench fever	Breakdown of public health measures
Plague	Economic development; land use
Diphtheria	Interruption of immunisation programme due to political changes
Tuberculosis	Human demographics and behaviour; industry and technology; international commerce and travel; breakdown of public health measures; microbial adaptation
Pertussis (whooping cough)	Refusal to vaccinate in some parts of the world because of the belief that injections or vaccines are not safe
Salmonella (food poisoning)	Industry and technology; human demographics and behaviour; microbial adaptation; food changes
E.coli O157	Food processing and shipment
Pneumoccus (pneumonia)	Human demographics; microbial adaptation; international travel and commerce; misuse and overuse of antibiotics
Cholera	Travel: a new strain (0139) apparently introduced to South America from Asia by ship, with spread facilitated by reduced water chlorination and also food

Figure 4.11 **Re-emerging infections 1980–2000 and factors contributing to their emergence**
(Source: ProMED wysiwyg://24/http;//sun00781.dn.net/promed/about/table3.html

- one third of the global population was infected with *Mycobacterium tuberculosis* bacillus
- 8 million new cases occur every year
- TB causes 2 million deaths each year.

LEDCs at risk?

The LEDCs in Africa and South East Asia are most at risk. Urbanisation and rapid population growth were two main factors, but the rapid rise of HIV/AIDS, which makes the sufferer far more likely to fall victim to TB, is the main culprit.

Transmission?

TB can be transmitted by **droplet infection** from saliva or from untreated milk from animals infected with the bovine form. The disease normally affects the lungs, filling them with tubercules which can destroy their structure (consumption). The sufferer loses weight, coughs up blood and has night sweats. The lungs can eventually collapse and the bacilli can spread throughout the bloodstream, and to organs such as the brain, or to the bones. It can remain dormant for several years.

Treatment?

The best form of treatment is **Directly Observed Therapy, Short-course (DOTS)**. This combines drug therapy with careful monitoring, which is essential. There is a phase using three different drugs, lasting two months. The second phase is important as it involves two drugs for four months, and prevents drug resistance.

Prevention?

The routine way of preventing TB in MEDCs is by the **BCG vaccine**, usually offered to children at puberty. The close contacts of an infected person are always examined and monitored carefully.

Why is it re-emerging and what is the threat in the UK?

Why are so many dying of a disease that is curable? The reasons are complex and irrefutably linked to Britain's underclass.... Those who live in cramped conditions and whose immune systems are suppressed are more likely to become sick and to infect others.

More than half the cases in Britain are among immigrants and refugees. In London, where the most detailed studies have been done, at least 50% of patients are unemployed, 5% have a history of homelessness, more than 7% are alcoholics and a further 7% are HIV+.

Catherine O'Brien, *The Times*, February 2001

Here is a picture similar to that in New York. In 1991 there was an epidemic there because: the USA was complacent about the threat; funding for clinics was cut; immunisation programmes were dropped.

In the late 1980s there was a sudden surge in cases; they trebled and 30% were **MDR (multi-drug resistant)**, as the TB would not respond to antibiotic treatment. It cost £40 billion to control.

In London 2.5% of TB cases are MDR-TB. The average TB case costs £6,000 to control. MDR-TB costs £60,000. Treatment lasts three times as long and must be completed. Failure to follow the treatment programme is the cause of MDR-TB in the first place. Patients feel so much better in the early stages of therapy that they often give up. The recommended ratio of nurses to patients is 1:50. In Newham, the London borough with the highest TB incidence, the ratio was 1:190. So £2 million more a year is needed (O'Brien 2001).

The TB hot spots in the UK are in cities with high numbers of immigrants – Birmingham, Bradford and Bolton. An outbreak occurred in Leicester in March 2001 in a school where 93% of the 1,200 pupils were Asian. It was the worst outbreak for 20 years. The origin of the disease was thought to be from a foreign trip (Wright 2001). Unfortunately, the BCG vaccine programme had been suspended in September 1999. In London it was re-introduced because of the large numbers of cases.

If TB can occur so easily in MEDCs then it can occur anywhere.

Tuberculosis has been described as the world traveller that does not need a visa.

Thomas Stuttaford, 'Rise of disease has links to the Empire',
The Times, April 2001

d) Methicillin-resistant *Staphylococcus aureus* (MRSA) re-emerges, along with others

This first came to prominence in the early 1940s, when staff at hospitals in MEDCs began to observe particularly vicious infections which did not respond to penicillin. They were often fatal; sufferers untreatable by conventional means and dying a lingering death as their systems gradually succumbed to infection. The diagram (Figure 4.12) shows how this process has been gradual, beginning with the discovery of penicillin itself. Since then other diseases have been found to resist penicillin too: the sexually transmitted disease (STD) gonorrhoea; TB; malaria; hepatitis B; typhoid; shigella dysentery; pneumonia; AIDS.

The causes of **resistance** (Heymann 2000) can be under-use of drugs in LEDCs. If patients cannot afford a full course they will take enough to kill off the weakest forms of the infection but will stop before the stronger forms have been destroyed fully. The wrong drug may be prescribed in many cases of mis-diagnosis. Careless practices

The discovery and loss of Penicillin in treating *Staphylococcus aureus*

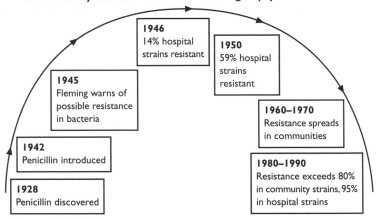

Figure 4.12 **The loss of penicillin and the emergence of MRSA**
(Source: WHO)

in LEDC hospitals are also to blame. Over-use of **antibiotics** for every small ailment and in food production is having the same effect in MEDCs. There is some hope that the situation will improve, as Japanese researchers are working on the genetic code for MRSA, and scientists at the University of East London have found allicin (a substance derived from garlic) effective in laboratory trials.

e) Ebola virus: a new haemorrhagic fever

What is it?

Ebola is an often-fatal disease caused by an RNA virus from the newly discovered **filoviridae** family. There are three sub-types, all of which cause haemorrhagic (heavy loss of blood) fevers. It was discovered in 1976, near the Ebola River in what is now the Democratic Republic of the Congo.

What are its symptoms?

The sufferer begins with a high fever, headache, muscle pains, sore throat, and diarrhoea and vomiting. After a week, bleeding from all body cavities begins; **multiple organ failure** follows fast as each is literally destroyed and liquefied by the virus. Death is usual, although some recover.

How did it originate?

The origin of the virus is unknown. One explanation is that it came from eating infected 'bush meat' (derived from monkeys in the rain forest). Certainly similar viruses exist in the monkey population in this part of Central Africa. Humans do not carry the virus, but an individual starts the transmission process after possible infection as above. This is then passed on by poor clinical practice in hospital, such as a neglect of 'barrier' nursing or not using sterile needles (**nosocomial infection**). The ritual embalming practice after death, common in the areas of Africa where Ebola is endemic, involves washing out all the body cavities. Since the virus is in the blood and faeces this is the other potent source of infection.

What geographical factors influence its incidence and spread?
The basic cause of new viruses such as Ebola lies in the mismanagement of the environment leading to a disturbance of the natural ecological balance. High population densities encourage deforestation and the desire to open up new roads through the rain forest means that new food sources become available to hunters, who take these to the nearest town. Monkey 'bush meat' is one such new food.

Where does it occur?
Outbreaks have been mainly in LEDCs in central Africa: Sudan, the Democratic Republic of the Congo (formerly Zaire), the Ivory Coast and Gabon. In Uganda there was a death rate of over 60% in the 2001 outbreak.

Is there a cure?
No cure exists at present. The best care is, therefore, supportive therapy after the patient has been isolated. The fluid and electrolyte balance must be carefully maintained. There are attempts to inject the victim with plasma from convalescent patients, but this is not a proven method. It is not considered necessary to commit funds for research as the disease is confined to a small number of LEDCs.

What are the social effects of the disease?
With a high death rate (up to 90% in some outbreaks) the most direct impact is the death of essential health workers. This is very likely, given the low levels of equipment and hygiene in many LEDC hospitals. Since the standard practice in African hospitals is for the patient's family to move in to provide food and some nursing care, family members are also potential victims. Catching the virus is all the more likely for the women who embalm the body as they have to wash it thoroughly first, thereby coming into contact with blood and faeces.

Another hazard might be the use of the virus as a component of **biochemical warfare**.

What are the economic effects?
The death of essential workers will obviously cause a decline in local healthcare standards. This will lessen the ability of the country to control and prevent any further outbreaks. Tourism could suffer if the

disease has been identified in areas where adventure holidays might be planned.

f) Bovine spongiform encephalopathy (BSE) and its new strain – vCJD

What are BSE and vCJD?
They are both from a class of diseases which affect chemical bundles called **prion proteins** which are found in the brain (*The Week* 2000). The healthy protein is somehow transformed into a form which changes the surrounding brain tissue into a useless spongy mass. Death is inevitable.

Is the disease new?
It was found in 1986 and is related to **scrapie**, which has long been known in sheep. The same type of condition has also been seen as **kuru** in Papua New Guinea when cannibalism led to the consumption of human brain tissue and in **CJD (Creutsfeld–Jakob disease)** in humans. It was thought that these diseases could not be transferred from one species to another.

Why did it spread so fast?
It seemed that BSE had been spread by recycling cattle remains in cattle feed. Perhaps there was a mutation in prion protein in a cow in south-west England creating the infection. Zoo animals and cats were found to be suffering from it. One theory (from scientists in New Zealand) is that the disease was imported with some antelope destined for a safari park.

When did it first occur in humans?
A new form of CJD began to emerge in the early 1990s. All the victims were teenagers: their brains had degenerated in the same way as those of the cattle with BSE. Hence a new strain of CJD was named – **new variant CJD,** or **vCJD**. Its cause is thought to be eating infected meat products. The reasons why younger people were involved was not known. Inherited susceptibility is another possibility. Those infected carried two copies of part of a gene linked to a specific amino-acid.

Is it really caused by infected beef?
In Britain, there has been a BSE epidemic among cattle and 85 of the known 86 cases of vCJD have occurred in Britain. France has had 126 BSE cases and Switzerland 138; Britain has had 12,732. A particular cluster of five victims appeared in the village of Queniborough in Leicestershire (Wright 2001). Here, the village butcher had used a traditional slaughter technique which involved inserting a rod into cows' brains to prevent the animals struggling. The animals slaugh-

tered by this technique were generally older than was usual – up to 30 months old, which increased the risk still further. All the meat in question was sold in the 1980s.

How many people are likely to die from vCJD?
A team of scientists from Oxford have put forward a projected total of 136,00 deaths, assuming an incubation period of 60 years. If the incubation period is below this then the total might be a few thousand.

Can people be screened for vCJD?
Post-mortem examination of the brain is the only sure way. Looking at tissue from the tonsils or from a brain scan might be helpful in diagnosis, but there is still no cure for vCJD.

Summary

1. Individuals experience morbidity (illness) in varying degrees of severity. These can range from mild or sub-clinical forms to acute (serious short-term illness) or chronic (long-term sickness) attacks.
2. The burden of disease refers to the effects on a society of illnesses in the population. This can be assessed by mortality (death) rates, incidence (the rates at which illness progresses) or by prevalence (the total number with that disease).
3. As countries move through the epidemiological transition, the burden of disease worldwide will shift so that 70% of deaths in LEDCs will be from non-infectious diseases by 2020.
4. The years lived with disability (YLDs), including mental illnesses, will be increasingly significant as populations age.
5. More research should be targeted on those conditions which add significantly to the global disease burden, for example pneumonia and diarrhoea.
6. HIV/AIDS is now a pandemic (worldwide). It is the human immunodeficiency virus which causes acquired immunodeficiency syndrome. It is thought to have originated in central Africa. International travel and IDU in addition to the upheaval of urbanisation have caused its rapid spread.
7. It has two main clades (types). The one found in Africa, spread mainly by heterosexual contact, is more infectious. These spread through unprotected sex, IDU with dirty needles, transfusion with contaminated blood and from mother to child in the womb.
8. The pattern of spread is often hierarchical diffusion along highways form large cities and other centres into rural areas.
9. Although expensive triple drug therapy is an option to prolong life in MEDCs, AIDS awareness education is the best option in LEDCs, which lack resources.
10. New Zealand, the Russian Federation, Thailand, Myanmar and South Africa are case studies illustrating a range of responses to HIV/AIDS.

11. Sleeping sickness is a parasite transmitted by the tsetse fly in central Africa. It was spread by the opening up of the forest areas by white settlers. Despite elimination programmes in the 1960s, it has returned, owing to conflict and civil war in the areas where it is endemic. It is often fatal and inflicts a heavy burden of disease in lost working years and lack of agricultural productivity. Depopulation of large areas can occur. Drug therapy is painful and expensive.

12. The ultimate aim of control strategies for all infectious diseases is to eradicate them completely from the planet. This has already occurred with smallpox. This can be done by imposing geographical barriers – by isolation and by quarantine. Immunity can be conferred by immunisation with vaccines.

13. Polio and measles are both targeted for eradication but difficulties with different types of virus, the timing of mass vaccinations and uncertainty about side effects have delayed plans so far. A falling take-up of vaccination means that the virus can become endemic once more.

14. Emerging and re-emerging diseases are those infectious diseases which may have only just come to light or those which have become more virulent for some reason. Factors such as land use changes – deforestation, irrigation, agricultural intensification and urbanisation, together with globalisation and the industrialisation of food production have encouraged this process.

15. Tuberculosis (TB) is one such disease. One third of the global population is infected, with Africa and South East Asia most at risk, especially where HIV/AIDS lowers the immunity of the population. In MEDCs, the main victims are often homeless, alcoholic drug users suffering from HIV/AIDS. New York had an epidemic in the 1980s. With a decline in BCG vaccination and the advent of MDR (multi-drug resistant) TB owing to incomplete therapy uptake, the disease is far more common.

16. MRSA (Methicillin-resistant *Staphylococcus aureus*) is a worrying development in the gradual decline in the effectiveness of antibiotics which has been happening ever since penicillin was discovered. Many other infections have since become resistant to it including malaria, typhoid and pneumonia. This can be explained by its under-use in LEDCs (failure to complete courses) and its over-use in MEDCs, which leads to weakened immune systems.

17. Ebola virus was discovered in 1976 in central Africa. It is a new type of virus, which causes extensive bleeding and destruction of internal organs and has no cure besides barrier nursing and fluid replacement. Mortality rates can be as high as 90%. It is thought to have been caused by eating monkey meat from hitherto remote areas of the forest. The appalling hygiene conditions in many central hospitals and the ritual embalming of corpses by women add to its spread, even though it is not a droplet infection.

18. vCJD (new variant CJD) is related to the brain disease BSE (bovine spongiform encephalopathy) found in cattle, the so-called 'mad cow' disease. It is a fatal human brain disease in which rogue proteins grow in the brain, turning it into a spongy mass. BSE emerged as the result of giving

cattle feed containing cattle remains and probably originated with antelope imported for a UK safari park. From the early 1990s, vCJD was
found especially in people under 25. There have been 86 cases, 85 of
which have been in the UK. It is thought that there will be thousands
more infected; the incubation period can be 20 to 30 years.

Suggested essay or report title

Discuss how and why disease and infection can have different impacts on a range of societies and communities.

General hints on writing essays and reports are to be found at the end
of Chapter 2.

Choice of title

- The command word 'discuss' means that you must take a wide-ranging
  look at the topic from a number of different viewpoints.
- Disease implies that degenerative (non-communicable) illnesses are
  included in addition to all types of infections. 'Societies' implies that you are
  looking at groups of people sharing common ideas and territory.
  'Communities' are smaller groups within society as a whole, such as the
  gay community in the USA or the black community in London.
- The theories and models behind this question are morbidity and mortality rates, the epidemiological transition (which will predict what types
  of diseases are likely to be found and where), the burden of disease
  (which estimates the – mainly economic – impact of illness on a community), dependency ratios (which look at the burden of care on different sectors of the population) and transmission models (which need to
  be understood if eradication is to take place).

Research

- Make a copy of the relevant parts of the chart (Frontispiece I) showing
  the outline for this chapter on to A3 paper.
- The choice must be balanced: infections in LEDCs (and emergent and re-
  emergent diseases in MEDCs) must be set against the degenerative diseases of the ageing societies in MEDCs.
- Your choice of case studies should reflect this balance.
- Mental illnesses are important in all areas and must not be forgotten.
- The how suggests that you must find details about the disease or infection and the why suggests that you look carefully at different impacts
  (social/economic/environmental).

Planning

- Drawing in all the links on your chart between theory and case study is
  important here.
- One of the main distinctions which must be made is between:
  - LEDCs where infectious diseases are the main cause of morbidity

and mortality and where those affected are still in the working population. The dependency ratio is thus made far less favourable as there are many orphans (especially with AIDS deaths). These are mainly agricultural societies where there is subsistence farming. . .and

- MEDCs where the main causes of morbidity and later mortality are the degenerative diseases in the ageing population, which makes the dependency ratio far less favourable as there are correspondingly fewer people in the working population to support those over retirement age. These are mainly sophisticated societies where there is a higher standard of living.

- Attempts to lessen the impacts must be considered, such as prevention and eradication for the infections, and careful planning for independence with adequate support for the degenerative diseases.
- The choice of case study should be at minimum two infections (HIV/AIDS should be one, with cholera or sleeping sickness or measles) and two degenerative diseases (for instance, Alzheimer's or cancer or heart disease), chosen because of the contrasts between them.
- The areas of study of these diseases should be in contrasting societies, for example New Zealand and South Africa or Canada and Nigeria.
- The concluding ideas will need to be carefully organised because there are so many issues to address.

Annotated maps, population pyramids and spider diagrams should be drawn to illustrate what you are going to discuss.

Geography's role in analysing the future challenges to health, welfare and societies

Geography provides an insight into the way in which individual societies respond to health and welfare challenges by identifying the underlying social and economic factors. It also helps in the **spatial analysis** of demand for healthcare and welfare. Through examining **demographic** (population) change rates, geography can help in **future resource planning**.

1 Funding healthcare

a) Different sources of funding; composition of health spend

What is a health system?

According to the World Health Organisation (WHO) Report 2000, a **health system** includes 'all the activities whose primary purpose is to promote, restore or maintain health'.

In the last 100 years, healthcare systems have evolved from informal family and small-scale private or charitable care into large and complex organisations. Germany first introduced state insurance for health service cover in 1883, followed by Belgium in 1894 and by Norway 15 years later. After the Revolution in 1917, universal state care was brought in by Russia. Japan and Chile also began insurance systems in the 1920s. In the UK, the National Health Service was launched in 1948. This offered free healthcare to all, financed through the taxation system. Former European colonies such as India had a health service exclusively for the urban elite. With independence in 1947, health improvement took its place in a series of Five-year Plans, with heavy state participation.

In what ways are health systems funded?

In the early twenty-first century, healthcare spending takes around 8% of world GDP, by comparison with 1948 where the figure was 3%. Systems have many sources of funding, locally, nationally and globally for example:

a. from taxation
b. from state social insurance schemes
c. from employers' contributions to workers' insurance schemes
d. from charitable sources and foundations
e. from private health insurance schemes

f.   from the patient's pocket (direct payments)
g.   from NGOs such as Oxfam and UNICEF and other sources of aid.

Each of these methods has its drawbacks. If an individual contributes by way of a **salary-related scheme** (c above), the contributions are related to what is earned. If an individual contributes by way of a private insurance scheme (e above), the amount is related to the health of that individual and the size of the risk it presents. Given the choice between these two methods, as was the case in Chile, those in the population who were in less good health chose to have their contributions related to their salary levels, rather than to pay highly for private health insurance.

In the case of **taxation, state social security schemes** and **contributions from salaries** (a, b and c), the risks are spread. A private individual has to meet his or her own risks with private health insurance. Thus a fit 35-year-old contributing in categories a, b or d, c above will be subsidising a 75-year-old's hip replacement. This **pooling mechanism** and **cross-subsidy** ensures the fairer distribution of healthcare. Through private medical insurance (e), that chronically sick 75-year-old would be paying out far more than the fit 35-year-old, who would not usually see any benefits from the contributions for many years.

Those most at risk, however, are those living in poverty in LEDCs where the only option is to **pay directly** for any service that they might receive (f above). This type of payment represents over 40% of the spending on healthcare in LEDCs. Unfortunately, any attempts to finance healthcare by general taxation (a above) are also difficult. LEDC taxation systems are notoriously inefficient, representing less than 20% of GDP on average. By contrast, 40% of the GDP of MEDCs is derived from taxation.

The WHO 2000 Report recommends that funding sources should be balanced carefully to ensure that they fulfil the following criteria for success:

• they should improve the population's health
• they should respond to expectations
• they should provide financial protection against the costs of ill health.

The 1999 WHO Report had identified the two major challenges confronting all systems as:

• ensuring efficiency
• achieving and maintaining universal coverage.

This means that health spending should be increased in order to alleviate the sufferings of the poorest in society:

in any country, the greatest burden of ill-health and the biggest risk of avoidable morbidity or mortality is borne by the poor ... the distribution of services in most countries remains highly skewed in favour of the better-off. The least organised and most inequitable may be paying for healthcare as an out-of-pocket basis...the financing burden falls disproportionately on the poorest...in trying to but health from their own pockets sometimes they only succeed in lining the pockets of others.

WHO Report 2000

b) Providing healthcare

Thus, the WHO recommended a '**new universalism**' of primary healthcare (provided by community-based medicine, for example General Practitioners), as opposed to secondary care (in hospitals). Figure 5.1 shows this concept.

What health needs and demands does a society have?

One of the traditional ways of providing healthcare was to estimate the needs of a society. This has often failed to satisfy its demands, as the poor, for instance, are often unable to voice their requirements. The difficulties of transport or of obtaining compensation for time lost at work can, for example, have a bearing on whether to seek healthcare or not. One solution is to let funding follow the patient.

The Alma Ata conference, called by WHO in 1978, recommended that funding should be directed at meeting the basic needs of the poor such as providing adequate sanitation and clean water. This shows a drive to move into the next phases of the **epidemiological transition**, as the MEDCs have done. The poor, in particular, had primitive or

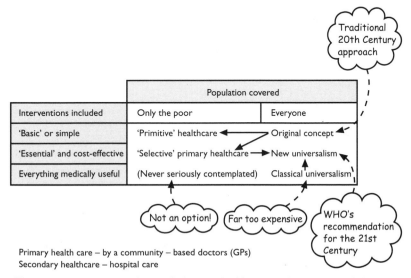

Primary health care – by a community – based doctors (GPs)
Secondary healthcare – hospital care

Figure 5.1 **Coverage of population and of interventions under different notions of primary healthcare**
(Source: WHO Report 2000)

non-existent primary care. The rich by-passed this, going straight to private care in hospital, and thus getting more from the system.

What resources exist for drug research and development?

In many LEDCs, especially **Highly Indebted Poor Countries (HIPCs)**, so much of the annual health budget is taken up with salaries that there are few resources left for research. Drugs developed by MEDC-based research laboratories (branded with specific trade names e.g. *Nurofen*) have had their patents jealously guarded so that the cheaper *generic* forms (with the pharmacological name e.g. *ibuprofen*) made in India, Thailand or Brazil could be substituted (Kennedy 2001).

It was argued by Oxfam (*The Week* 2001) that the five top drugs companies wield enormous power, having a combined worth of twice the GDP of sub-Saharan Africa and are conducting 'an undeclared drugs war against the world's poorest people'.

This is also especially devastating for those poor African countries ravaged by HIV/AIDS. A breakthrough occurred when a deal by Merck & Co and two other pharmaceutical companies was made with the government of the Ivory Coast, where 10% of the population was HIV positive. The agreement meant that the cost of HIV treatment was cut by 90%. Even so, the cost (between $500 and $600 per patient each year) is far above what the average LEDC spends on healthcare.

One global solution would be to tackle the AIDS problem as UNICEF has tackled mass vaccinations for measles, for example. Donor drugs companies could fund a programme for Africa at around $3 billion. *The Week* comments: 'not a high price, considering what is at stake'. Figure 5.2 summarises the situation.

Should poorer countries be given access to cheap generic drugs?

NO	YES
1. Unless controlled, the generic drugs business will inevitably undermine research and development into new drugs.	1. Millions die each year from preventable, treatable diseases. It is immoral to deny them access to the cheapest drugs.
2. The problem is poverty, not the high cost of patented drugs. Most poor nations can't even afford the cost of generic drugs.	2. Poor nations should not have to foot the bill for research and development into drugs aimed at richer nations.
3. The drugs industry is a commercial business not a charity. If we are to subsidise the poor, the taxpayer should foot the bill.	3. Allowing poorer countries to undercut patent medicine prices will have minimal effect on drugs industry profits.

Figure 5.2 **Should poorer countries be given access to cheap generic drugs?**
(Source: *The Week* 17 March 2001)

What human resources are needed?

It is also difficult to maintain an adequate supply of **human resources**. Medical personnel in MEDCs can be in short supply because of quotas imposed on medical courses, for instance. In addition, the low pay for nurses and ancillary workers and high cost of living in some prosperous areas lead to shortages. In LEDCs, often with formerly state-controlled service now subject to market forces with the decline in socialist funding systems, there is often a surplus of trained staff. International migration flows are increasingly redressing this balance.

It is estimated by WHO (2000) that 15% of all the physicians in Mexico are unemployed. In Thailand and South Africa there is a shortage, especially in rural areas. The breakdown of the old socialist system in the Russian Federation has lead to a surplus of doctors.

In the UK in the 1960s and 1970s, Commonwealth doctors were recruited in large numbers to fill primary care posts, often in inner cities where there are large ethnic minority communities. They frequently work as single-handed GPs and are in areas suffering multiple deprivation. As they approach retirement age there are doubts about finding replacements, despite government promises of increased numbers of medical school places becoming available. An extra 2,000 GPs have been promised but the British Medical Association (BMA) feels that at least 10,000 are needed. Cash incentives to encourage GPs to stay on after the age of 60 have also been introduced. (Hawkes 2001). An ageing society makes more demands on its doctors in any case; all MEDCs fit this pattern (see the second half of Chapter 5). A new contract in 2002 will not improve the morale of the 90% of GPs who indicated their opposition to it in a BMA questionnaire.

Jamaican nurses frequently migrate to the USA. The UK, too, had a doubling of applications from nurses overseas in 2001, with 1,000 a week being received (Charter 2001). Most new recruits came from the Philippines, South Africa, Eire and the West Indies. Nurses from these countries are drawn to the UK, as they are English speakers. British nurses correspondingly are attracted to better conditions in Australia and the USA; 5,000 applied for jobs overseas in 2000.

How is funding co-ordinated?

It is essential in the developing world to co-ordinate sources of funding in a **sector-wide approach (SWAP)** lest inappropriate provision is made, such as a 100-bed hospital in Sri Lanka financed by an aid project (g above), which was far too expensive to maintain technically.

The balance of government expenditure with other items, such as defence, is further detrimental to healthcare in LEDCs. Pakistan, for instance, spends a similar proportion of its GDP on health and on defence. (Japan spends seven times as much on its health service as it does on defence). In Figure 5.3 the **health spend mix** for 23 countries, selected from the WHO 2000 study of 191 countries, is shown. Here the balance of **public spending** (derived from taxes and state health

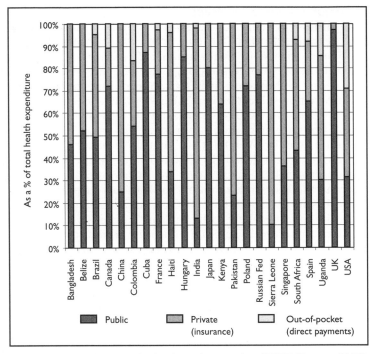

Figure 5.3 **Health spend of selected countries (WHO Report 2000)**

and social security schemes) is compared with the percentage of
private insurance spending and with **direct out-of-pocket spending**.
The contrasts between the UK, the USA and Sierra Leone, for
instance, are especially marked. The reasons behind these trends can
be found in the type of healthcare system in each country.

c) Field's model of healthcare types

One model which attempts to **classify health service types** is by Field
(1989) and is shown in Figure 5.4. The groupings emphasise the roles
of the individual doctor, any medical organisations to which he or she
might belong, the ownership of facilities such as clinics and medical
equipment, how the patient pays for healthcare and the influence of
the state in formulating healthcare policy. This model can be applied
to most healthcare systems and allows easy comparison.

Emergent healthcare – LEDCs

Tropical Africa

Is there any healthcare?
It has been estimated that over 200 million people in tropical Africa
were without access to health services in 1999 (Meade and Earickson

Type of healthcare	Main characteristics	Examples
EMERGENT	• Healthcare viewed as an item of personal consumption • Physician operates as a solo entrepreneur • Professional associations powerful • Private ownership of facilities • Direct payment to physicians • Minimal role in healthcare for the state	Bangladesh Belize Brazil Colombia Haiti India Kenya Pakistan Sierra Leone South Africa Uganda
PLURALISTIC	• Healthcare viewed mainly as a consumer good • Physician operated as a solo entrepreneur • Professional organisations very powerful • Private and public ownership of facilities • State's role in healthcare minimal and indirect	USA
INSURANCE/ SOCIAL SECURITY	• Healthcare as an insured/guaranteed consumer good or service • Physicians operate as solo entrepreneurs and as members of medical organisations • Professional organisations strong • Private and public ownership of facilities • Payment for services mostly indirect • State's role in healthcare central but indirect	France Japan Singapore Spain
NATIONAL HEALTH SERVICE	• Healthcare as a state supported service • Physicians operate as solo entrepreneurs and as members of medical organisations • Professional organisations fairly strong • Facilities mainly publicly owned • Payment for services indirect • State's role in health care central and direct	Canada UK
SOCIALISED	• Healthcare a state-provided public service • Physicians are state employed • Professional organisations weak or non-existent • Facilities wholly publicly owned • Payments for services entirely indirect • State's role in healthcare is total	China Cuba Hungary Poland Russian Fed

Figure 5.4 **Field's model of healthcare types**

2000). The average doctor:patient ratio was over 5,000:1. In MEDCs it is around 500:1.

How effective is it?

Outside cities, **traditional medicine** remains the norm. The 'healer' employs a wide range of psychosocial and dramatic means in addition to medication. Often the whole family or indeed the whole community is involved in the process. In many African countries healthcare is a mixture of traditional, modern, military, governmental and voluntary organisations. Large debts and externally imposed **structural adjustment policies** (SAPs) have further eroded health spending. Nations such as Gambia, Rwanda, Angola, Ethiopia and Sierra Leone have been ravaged by war, poverty and famine. Defence spending often figures more largely than any other claim on finances. Most of the medical care in this situation is in the hands of the military unless there is provision by charitable or international aid organisations.

This account of healthcare in Sierra Leone is typical:

> Sierra Leone had no medical school, so native physicians fell into two categories; the ones who were trained in the West and the ones who were trained in the Soviet Union. The doctors who'd attended medical school in the West, if they ever came back, generally found lucrative practices in Freetown, or else they worked for the government, gaining political points, a reasonable pension plan, and a bustling private practice in the afternoons and evenings. They rarely came up country.
>
> Most of the Soviet-trained physicians ...went into the government hospital system ...and were immediately dispatched into the rural areas ....The local hospital was filled with these inept doctors ...little better than butchers. They practised on the unsuspecting local population with little supervision, if any. It did not take long even for the most illiterate villagers to figure out that the local hospitals were to be avoided whenever possible.
>
> Unfortunately there was often nowhere else to go for help. In search of a reasonable, mission-run hospital, sick people in desperate condition would travel miles over terrible roads in little poda-podas, small blue pick-up trucks that functioned as all-purpose buses, usually crammed with people, produce and animals ...

Joseph McCormick and Susan Fisher-Hoch, *The Virus Hunters*, 1997

India

Is there any healthcare?

Two **traditional** types of medicine – ayurvedic and unani – still exist in the country. The healthcare is highly diversified; both western and traditional practitioners have private practices. Over 75% of India's 1 billion people live in rural areas but the vast majority of hospitals are to be found in the cities. In Mumbai (Bombay), Kolkata (Calcutta) and New Delhi in the mid-1980s, the doctor:patient ratios were 500:1. In the rural areas it was 7,000:1.

How effective is it?

India's **fertility rate** is still high (570 per 100,000 live births) and this contributes to the dilution of health services and their infrastructure. Its 3,700 urban centres and 600,000 villages are poorly served by ineffective health policies; many rural communities lack clinics and hospitals (Cassen et al 1999). In the southern state of Tamil Nadu the government has sponsored mobile clinics. The drawback is that they are poorly advertised and do not keep to schedules. The staff also need better training. There is an **integrated nutrition programme** in the state, which has gone some way to combating the undernourishment of children under 5 years old. It is estimated that 50% of young children in India are malnourished.

Nevertheless, the **epidemiological transition** is occurring which means that there is a rising incidence of **degenerative diseases**. An ageing population will need more geriatric medicine (Cassen 1999).

Supporting the Indian economy is a major part of the World Bank's outgoings; with loans of over $44 billion India is its largest borrower. Nonetheless, government spending on health has been as low as 1.5% of GDP, with public health coming off very badly. Any measures have been poorly executed, in addition. In the World Bank's opinion: 'the institutional base for health services is weak, nongovernmental services are under-utilised, and....The private sector is virtually completely unregulated and offers some of the worst – and the best – care ever seen.' Meade and Earickson (2000).

Pluralistic healthcare – the USA

How can a market economy deliver healthcare?

The United States is unique among MEDCs as its system is provided by 'a private market of thousands of independent doctors, pharmacies, clinics and so on...' (Meade and Earickson 2000). This means that the government has little influence in overall planning. In the 1960s, however, the Democrat government established the following systems:

- **Medicaid** – to provide medical care to the poor on state benefits;
- **Medicare** – which was similar provision for the elderly.

Payment is made for: out-patient treatment; doctors' fees; hospitalisation; surgery; equipment and appliances.

How effective is the system?

Costs have risen rapidly. The main reasons are: increased demand; separate payments to doctors and to hospitals preventing efficient integration; an ageing population needing expensive medical treatment; inflation and rising GNP.

Nonetheless, there is still a significant section of the population who are without adequate insurance cover – more than 44 million people.

In the mid-1970s, a series of health systems agencies (HSAs) were formed to be responsible for health planning for populations of around 2 million. The HSA boundaries fitted administrative boundaries as much as possible. There are still spatial imbalances, however.

What recent developments have there been?

1. **The Health Maintenance Organisation (HMO).** This is a system where subscribers pre-pay for medical care. Around 67 million people use this system, which involves doctors working efficiently in group practices. Obviously it discriminates against those of low income and with serious illnesses.

2. **Standardising Medicare payments.** These were formerly set by individual hospitals, which was very inefficient. As this represents 40% of hospital revenues, standardisation has helped reduce costs.

3. **Free-standing ambulatory surgery centers (FASCs).** These perform day surgery at a low cost.

4. **Managed care.** This is a recent – and controversial – move by insurance companies and larger HMOs to dictate to the medical care providers (doctors, hospitals, clinics, for instance) the amount and type of healthcare which they will fund. 'Disease management programmes show promise in improving the care of patients with chronic illnesses. But commercial disease management may have damaging unintended consequences for healthcare systems. Healthcare institutions should initiate in-house disease management programmes that assist primary care physicians in doing a better job...' (T. Bodenheimer 2000).

Insurance/social security – France

How does the system work?

French patients can chose their doctors, see them as often as they like, visit other doctors for second opinions, consult specialists at will, even check themselves in at hospitals. ...No rationing, no queues...

David Lawday, 'A hypochondriac's paradise (UK versus French health care system)', *New Statesman*, 18 September 1998

In 2000, the French health service was judged the most effective by WHO from a total of 191 different countries.

- It functions using the social security system, backed up for many people by private insurance schemes.
- The patient pays on the spot for medical care, which is then reimbursed. Up to 75% of the cost of treatment or medicines can be recovered.
- Extra private insurance from a mutual assurance company means that the rest of the outlay can be recovered and medicines are free.
- A recent innovation is a patient's 'smart card', which contains all this information and can be operated by whichever practitioner the patient is using.
- GPs are usually solo practitioners.
- The patient can chose to see any doctor as frequently as he or she would like.
- Hospital care and transport to and from the hospital is free for more serious diseases. Private hospital costs are reimbursable.
- Wards are always of two patients only.
- There is a scale of charges approved by the government.
- There are no waiting lists.
- There are 2.8 doctors per thousand citizens.

Are there any drawbacks?

There are some problems with this system, which the government is attempting to address:

- It is very expensive.
- The French spend about 10% of their GDP (which is larger than that of the UK anyway) on healthcare.
- The social security system which finances the health service is, in turn, run by a pay-as-you-earn tax scheme which takes 45% of the GDP.
- Employers pay 25% of wage bills in social security for their employees; this seriously damages the prospects of industrial and commercial growth.
- Health spending is fast getting out of control; it grew at 4.9% in the first half of 2000, which was twice the government's target figure of 2.5% ($92 billion). Hospital spending was, however, well within limits – but this led to thousands of bed closures.
- Doctors' earnings depend on their 'custom'; money goes direct to their pockets from the patient but there are schemes to reduce fees if they seem to be in excess, for example cardiologists must now charge less for visits.
- There is no interest in limiting the care provided by a doctor at the moment but a system using referral to specialists by GPs (as in the UK) is planned.
- Despite being reimbursed 100% of costs, those on low incomes had, until the invention of the smart card, to find money for the consultation in the first place.
- Health dispensaries are the unsatisfactory alternative for those too poor to seek a doctor's advice.

- The quality of hospital treatment varies widely.
- Preventive care (for example, vaccination and screening) is poor.

National Health Service

The UK

How did it start?

The UK Labour government led the world in the foundation of a free National Health Service in 1948. Its founder Aneurin Bevan was determined to make good health a priority for all citizens: 'The essence of a satisfactory health service is that rich and poor are treated alike.'

Its main aims were:

1. to meet all acute and chronic (emergency and long-term) medical needs
2. to make healthcare free and universal
3. to fund the system from general taxation
4. to give groups of doctors professional independence.

What was it like before the NHS?

To give some idea of the changes that ordinary citizens experienced in 1948, this is an account of the village surgery in Twyford, near Winchester, in Hampshire:

In the early days the doctors made their own medicines. Dr Thomas Roberts grew a supply of foxgloves in his garden to provide digitalis. He ground up the leaves and dissolved them in alcohol to treat his heart patients. He died in 1887. A child with diphtheria coughed straight in his face. There were no antibiotics and the disease was a killer ....

In the twenties the doctors did their own minor surgery. One afternoon a week the doctor removed children's tonsils in the Parish Hall. There is the well-known story of two small children who walked down from Hazeley cottages, clutching their sixpences (2.5p) for the doctor. They had their tonsils removed and then walked back.

Doctors made many more home visits than they do today. This helped limit the spread of infection. They were still expected to attend morning and evening surgery no matter how many visits they had made. There was no system of appointments; patients arrived as early as they could and were dealt with in turn. On some occasions surgery could go on until 9 or 10 o'clock at night.

Paying for the doctor was always a worry for poor people. Most working men paid into a friendly society which then covered their medical expenses. In 1899 Dr George Roberts formed a Club for the wives and families of working men. They paid 3d (around 1p) a week which entitled them to free treatment and medicine . . . .

Private patients formed the bulk of the doctor's income. The usual fee for a visit was one guinea (£1.05), and had been for 30 years. The money was often left discreetly beside the doctor's hat on the hallstand. Clergymen and doctor's widows were not charged. Often debts mounted up and there was little hope of them being paid. Some attempted to pay in kind and the doctor would find eggs or vegetables left in his car . . . .The old and infirm were sent to the old Workhouse Infirmary.

All this changed with the National Health Service. Everyone had to be assigned to a doctor's list and he received 12/- (60p) a year for each patient. Treatment, medicine, eye tests and glasses, and dental treatment were all free and doctors were inundated with requests for anything and everything, from reading glasses to aspirin, from new dentures to cotton wool.

Doreen Pearce and Stanley Crooks, *Twyford – Ringing the Changes*, George Mann, Winchester 1999

How has the situation changed since 1948?

There have been profound changes in the NHS since 1948. What was designed to eliminate ill health has now become increasingly inefficient at delivering healthcare for all. Some of the main reasons are:

- increasing patient expectations
- the development of many more medical interventions and drugs, for example heart transplants and fertility treatment
- longer life expectancy
- complex and wasteful administration and deployment of resources, with little monitoring
- a vast range of medical specialties and support services
- fewer but larger and more sophisticated hospitals
- the elimination of easily cured infectious diseases (with antibiotics) and their replacement with difficult-to-treat degenerative conditions such as cancer, heart disease and Alzheimer's, as the epidemiological transition would predict.

Successive governments have found that the NHS has become difficult to manage. What was once the envy of the world has been undergoing a series of very necessary reforms. It is becoming clear that Bevan's vision is impossible in today's world. 'The concept of the NHS as a comprehensive service may have outlived its usefulness' according to a BMA report. (Charter 2001)

What government action has there been?

The latest developments in NHS Reform are the White Paper of 1999, which was followed by The NHS Plan in July 2000. The previous Conservative government had allowed an element of funding freedom for certain GPs' practices but there was criticism that this favoured more efficient practices in middle-class areas. Since these could effectively refer and fund patients to any hospital they chose, it meant that those poorer inner-city practices were further disadvantaged. A so-called 'two-tier' health service resulted. It was this that the Labour government reforms of 1999 and 2000 were seeking to eliminate, for example by the formation of **Health Action Zones (HAZs)**.

All primary health workers were to be linked in **Primary Care Groups** of 50 GPs or more (Figure 5.5). These would, in time, become freestanding Trusts and would buy services from **Hospital Trusts**. This replaced **Health Authorities** and allowed more local decision-making by providers. Associated with these changes came a system of regulation including healthcare initiatives and rewards, increased use of IT, quality controls on a local and national scale, and NHS Direct (a medical helpline).

The NHS Plan in 2000 (NHS 2000) proposed changes to deal with the time patients had to wait to see consultants and to have surgery (Figure 5.6). More resources were to be made available and targets were set for improvements to all aspects of the service but, at the same time, doubts were raised about funding, which represented an increase of 6.3%.

What is it like in practice?
The effects of the new system can be seen in the way in which primary care is organised in Mid-Hampshire (which includes the village surgery in Twyford). The map (Figure 5.7) shows the **PCT (Primary Care Trust)** area, which stretches from Andover in the north-west to Winchester and southwards to the outskirts of Portsmouth. It has a population of approximately 120,000, of which about 10,000 are over 74 years of age. Although the area is essentially typical of a southern 'shire' county there are variations in the need for healthcare as shown by the **Jarman scores**. Rural dwellers are essential car users, so this factor cannot easily predict social status. In addition, middle-class patients 'use' their GP more frequently, which means that any funding alloction is distorted.

There is one main hospital in Winchester – the Royal Hampshire County Hospital – run by the Winchester and Eastleigh Healthcare Trust. There is also a small private hospital in Winchester. Andover has a Community Hospital which will be taken over by the PCT.

The greatest concentration of need in the Winchester area (Figure 5.8) is in local authority estates and in the older housing near the centre where there are many elderly people living alone. Nearly one in five of those in the north of the city are aged over 74 and in five other wards 10% of the population is over 74. The three city practices are large and have mean list sizes of 1,854 per doctor (UK average

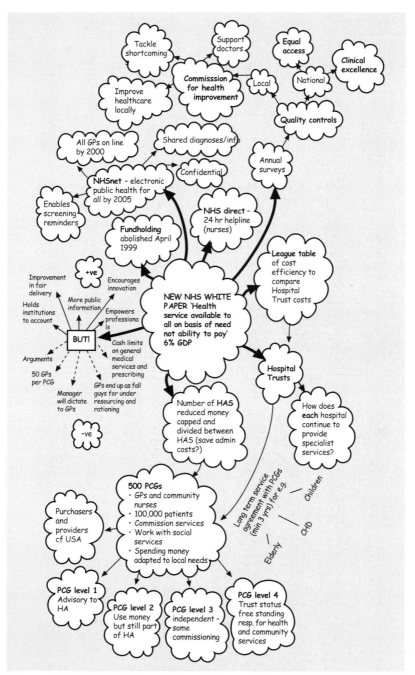

Figure 5.5 **NHS White Paper diagram**
(Source: NHS white paper 1999)

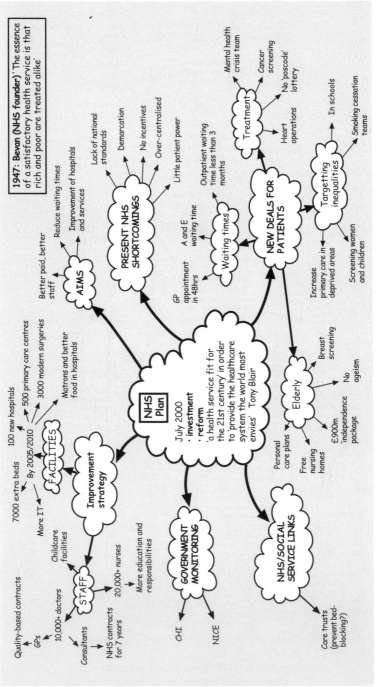

Figure 5.6 **NHS plan 2000 diagram**
(Source: NHSplan 2000)

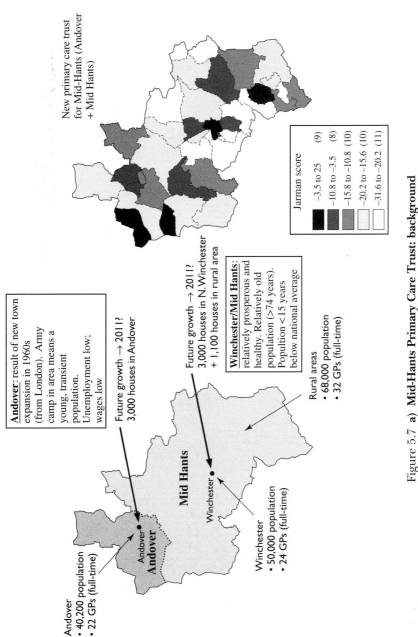

Andover: result of new town expansion in 1960s (from London). Army camp in area means a young, transient population. Unemployment low; wages low

Future growth → 2011? 3,000 houses in Andover

Future growth → 2011? 3,000 houses in N.Winchester + 1,100 houses in rural area

Winchester/Mid Hants: relatively prosperous and healthy. Relatively old population (>74 years). Population <15 years below national average

Rural areas
• 68,000 population
• 32 GPs (full-time)

Andover
• 40,200 population
• 22 GPs (full-time)

Andover

Mid Hants

Winchester

Winchester
• 50,000 population
• 24 GPs (full-time)

New primary care trust for Mid-Hants (Andover + Mid Hants)

Jarman score

	−3.5 to 25	(9)
	−10.8 to −3.5	(8)
	−15.8 to −10.8	(10)
	−20.2 to −15.6	(10)
	−31.6 to −20.2	(11)

Figure 5.7 a) **Mid-Hants Primary Care Trust: background**
b) **Mid-Hants Primary Care Trust 1991 Jarman Underprivileged Area Score by Electoral Ward**
(Source: Mid-Hants Primary Care Trust)

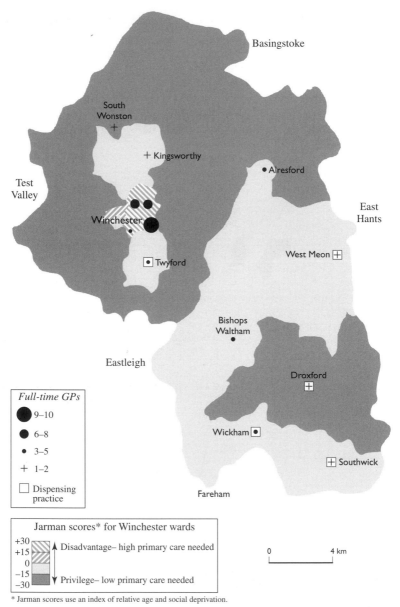

Figure 5.8 **Map of Winchester District (part of Mid-Hants Primary Care Trust) showing Jarman Scores and GP provision**
(Source: ibid)

2,100). The funding allocation of one of them, St Clements Partnership, was £256,795 for 2000–1.

The trust's guiding principle is 'to address inequalities and improve the health of our communities'. The following schemes are underway:

1. preventing falls in the elderly
2. reducing coronary heart disease in those under 75 (the ALIVE project) – the SMR from CHD has fallen from 160/100,000 in 1989 to 105 in 1999. The target is 40% reduction by 2010.
3. promoting back care
4. integrating mental health and learning disability teams
5. offering extra help to vulnerable families
6. working in collaboration with social workers to help older people and those in Winchester prison
7. taking patients' views into account.

Each practice has a number of targets to be attained in order to obtain extra funding, such as reducing the prescription of expensive anti-ulcer drugs and substituting their generic equivalent. The target date for all practices to be on NHS net computer network was 1 April 2001.

The future planning of healthcare must address a number of issues, such as the supply of GPs. Figure 5.9 shows that there will be a need to recruit a large number soon, as more than half are over 45. Of the younger doctors there is a predominance of female partners, which is a general trend in medicine as a whole. There will be an 8% growth in those over 74, which will put extra demands on the service by 2004. The South East has to provide a large number of new houses in the next decade and plans have also to address the projection of 3,000 new households in the north of Winchester, as mentioned in the 2001–2011 Structure Plan. It is calculated that there should be three new GPs for every 2,000 new houses.

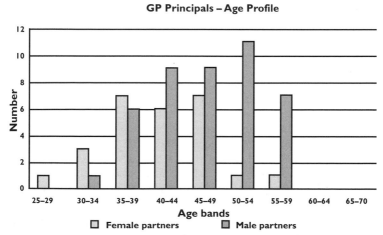

Figure 5.9 **The Mid-Hants PCG (Winchester area) GP principals age profile**
(Source: ibid)

Can the system survive?
Doubts were expressed from many quarters over the likely success of the reforms. Ian Bogle, chairman of the BMA (*The Week* 2000) commented that 'we need more doctors, more nurses and more beds ...'

If NHS Plan targets are met, the UK will have 1.7 doctors per 1,000 people. However, Germany has long had 3.4 and Greece 4 per 1,000. The improvements to the workforce will be very costly. Total health spending has risen from £40.8 billion in 1997 to £69 billion in 2000 (Miles et al 2001). Suggestions as to how to fund it were made by the Fabian Society (Brittan 2000), which proposed a tax specifically identified for health, or the use of the proceeds from VAT or National Insurance contributions.

> We are still fixated by the belief that the government should pay for health treatment and run the hospitals. Why can't we ever learn from the successful mix of private and public medicine used by such countries as France, Germany and the US? Taxes only finance a small proportion of their GDP on health than Britain ....Standards are correspondingly higher, even in America ....In most areas, our government is proud to commission studies into how other nations conduct their business. 'Why is the Department of Health so obstinate?'
>
> Andrew Alexander, 2000

> It's time we faced up to some uncomfortable facts about the Health Service ...We have become terribly spoilt. The developed world spends about 70 times as much on health as poorer countries; and because we can afford to pay high prices, pharmaceutical companies concentrate almost all their efforts on 'quality of life' drugs for the rich nations, instead of treating major tropical killers. If we genuinely believe that healthcare is an issue of human rights and equality we had better start demanding a lot less of it.
>
> John Humphrys, 2001

What is the role of private health care?
It was suggested that **acute services**, which make the NHS much more expensive than the **planned (elective) care** offered by the private sector, could make use of private hospital beds. More than 12 million people in the UK have private healthcare in any case (Doyle et al 2000). In 2000, the NHS spent £1.2 billion on healthcare from the private sector (Charter 2001); the private provider BUPA treated 1,373 NHS patients in the last quarter of 2000.

Private health organisations offer a quick and efficient service to those who can pay insurance premiums, which are often provided by their employers. The PPP organisation pays around £1.6 million in treatment costs every working day. Its brochure lists the following advantages of using its system: immediate access to hospital treatment; help and information whenever it is needed; individual specialist attention; annual eye test; two-yearly health check. A patient comments: 'I am indebted to you for saving me from the debilitating effect of a long wait and making it possible to be treated with the maximum of comfort and speed.' Ever-lengthening NHS **waiting lists,** with nearly 400,000 waiting more than 13 weeks for a first consultation and measured in years not months for some conditions such as hip replacements, are a big factor. The desire to keep NHS hospital beds at full capacity, reducing the numbers from 163,000 in 1990 to 134,923 in 2000 (thus allowing no 'slack' for emergencies such as winter 'flu epidemics) has also fuelled the desire for private healthcare. While the NHS deals with **acute** situations such as fractures and heart attacks reasonably efficiently, **elective surgery** is in a poor state.

What role is played by charities?

The role of charitable organisations is to offer support in a variety of situations not covered by the NHS. There is a wide range, some concentrating as much on welfare as on health. The main types are (see Figure 5.10):

* those linked to giving information and help for specific conditions, such as The Down's Syndrome Association or The Terence Higgins Trust (HIV/AIDS)
* those which offer support to patients and their families through their own staff, such as MacMillan Cancer Nurses
* those which provide mainly in-patient care, such as the hospice movement
* those which maintain extra services in NHS institutions like selling newspapers or providing transport for out-patient appointments, such as The League of Hospital Friends
* those which provide for the overall health and welfare of, for example, drug addicts or the homeless, such as Shelter, or the elderly, such as Age Concern.

The workers in all these organisations, some of whom have experienced the same problems as those they try to help, are a very necessary part of the total provision of health and welfare in the UK. Many of them are volunteers, which makes their work doubly valuable.

Canada

How does the system work?

Canada's aim was always to provide its citizens with equal access to healthcare regardless of their ability to pay. Its ten provinces, however, each had their own method of delivery. In 1971 the system known as **Medicare** came into being. This provided comprehensive coverage, allowing patients to take their benefits with them from one province to another. It was available to all permanent residents on uniform terms.

The Down's Syndrome Association offers help and support for those people with this congenital condition, which creates learning difficulties and medical conditions such as heart disease. It promotes a positive image with local groups. It funds research, such as giving £255,843 to investigating the link between Down's and Alzheimer's disease.

The Terrence Higgins Trust helped 9,500 people with HIV/AIDS in 2000. It is Europe's largest AIDS charity and is funded by grant aid from the EU and the UK Department of Health and by donations. It has a 24-hour AIDS help line. It not only provides support but is also instrumental in health education for groups such as gay men, who are especially at risk.

Naomi House is a hospice in Hampshire providing terminal care for children drawn from the whole of central Southern England. It has 50 staff but can only take a small number of children as each needs intensive nursing care. Families are also accommodated and respite care is used too. Running the hospice costs £300 per family per day, which means that £1 million a year is needed.

Shelter began in 1966 in London in response to a television programme about homelessness. It now operates all over the UK and had an income of £20 million in 1999, of which £11.9 million came as donations, and £3.9 million was in the form of grants. Its main aim is to fight homelessness and the practice of putting homeless people into expensive but highly ineffective bed-and-breakfast accommodation. It also enables such people to have access to healthcare, which would otherwise be very difficult to obtain.

Age Concern is an organisation which strives to get the best in life for people over 55 years of age. Problems addressed are as varied as assisting with income, housing and long-term care difficulties. It is working to help those who are house bound and has 250,000 volunteers in the UK. In 1999–2000 it had an income of £28.2 million of which nearly one third came from fund-raising.

Figure 5.10 **Examples of charities providing health and welfare support in the UK**
(Sources: charity websites)

This system provided care for a great deal less per patient than in the USA. Nonetheless, it became increasingly expensive throughout the 1980s and 1990s. Funding for the system and for education and social services was put under pressure by government debt. In addition, those with low incomes and in rural areas were under-served. This was especially true of the **indigenous groups** (First Nations and Inuit). Programmes to allow these groups to have control over their own healthcare are growing. There is also a non-insured benefits scheme for those unable to obtain drugs and medical supplies (Health Canada 2000).

Can it be cost-effective?
The problem for the Canadian government lay in trying to fund universal care while balancing its budget. At the same time, physicians wanted to retain professional freedom while consumers wanted a choice of providers.

These measures accompanied a wave of hospital cuts and closures which has been difficult to implement (Meade and Earickson 2000). Seven hospitals in Montreal were closed in the late 1990s; primary care was unable to respond to the increased need. The five teaching hospitals were linked to form a 'super hospital' (Pulanic 1999). Another example of the expensive duplication of resources is possibly the 'walk-in' primary medical centre found in urban areas (Jones 2000). There are no plans to abolish them, however. Walk-in centres:

- are not connected to a hospital
- are open for extended hours
- accept patients without appointment or referral
- are used by predominantly female patients (68%)
- tend to deal with patients under 35 and children with minor medical conditions
- refer very few patients (4%) on to hospital
- are under-used by the elderly and chronically sick
- are viewed by some sceptics as 'McDonald's medicine'
- do not always link effectively with the patient's general practitioner.

In September 2000 the First Ministers of the provincial governments resolved to

1. reform primary care, especially as an alternative to expensive emergency departments
2. make prescribing more cost effective
3. improve system performance by careful monitoring (CICS 2000).

An increase in funding of $15.6 billion was announced to restore some of the cuts in the Medicare system, but it was evident that demand would continue to be high. Moreover, the provincial governments had the option of diverting some of the funds to higher education and social services.

The Canadian Medical Association's survey at the time showed, however, that 80% of Canadians rated access to affordable and high-quality healthcare first among public spending programmes (Spurgeon 2000).

How does the service work in the remote areas?

In Yukon Province, for instance, there are four incentives available to induce medical professionals to work in such a remote and sparsely populated area (Figure 5.11): a progressive healthcare environment; a diverse range of practice types; a variety of healthcare initiatives; a fee rate 50% higher than in other provinces.

It is difficult to see how health services for this population can be further streamlined in view of the great distances involved.

Socialised

Cuba

Is it possible to offer high quality healthcare to all with few resources?
Cuba's health service is remarkably effective whichever way it is assessed.

- In the WHO table Cuba ranked 39th out of 191 countries.
- The USA ranks 37th but spends $1,193 per head on health as opposed to $109 in Cuba.
- Cuba has the highest **life expectancy** in the Caribbean (75 years compared with a mean of 57).
- In spite of having the lowest GDP in Latin America Cuba cut its IMR from 60/1,000 in 1954 to 7.9/1,000 in 1996 (half the figure for Washington DC).
- Cuba has the highest survival rate for children under five in the world when its GNP is taken into account (Kirkpatrick 2000).
- Cuba spends a high proportion of its budget on primary and preventive healthcare.
- For a population of 11 million there are 30,000 family doctors (*consultarios*).
- By the end of 2001 the goal is 66,000 doctors (giving a ratio of 170:1) and 10,000 dentists, with an increase in the number of home-birth units. This service is free on demand.
- Community nurses make fortnightly visits to infants under 1 year old and monitor those with hypertension on a daily basis, and advise on lifestyle changes.
- Secondary care consists of 442 polyclinics, 272 hospitals, 4 new mental health centres and research institutes.
- The new goals for the health service in 2000 were to improve mobile medical assistance (compare the USA) to reduce hospital bed demand for less serious cases.

Cuba's economy is based on sugar cane exports (60% of foreign earnings) and tourism. In 1920, around two-thirds of the agricultural land was owned by US companies. In 1959, a guerrilla campaign led by Fidel Castro expelled the US companies and nationalised their assets. The favoured trading partner became the former Soviet Union but, since 1990, the economy has been in decline. In 1992, the USA placed an embargo on food imports. This resulted in over 50,000 cases of malnutrition, with all the neurological diseases associated with famine, for instance eye damage, deafness and pain in hands and feet. In addition to the food import restrictions there are no basic drugs to treat, for example, heart disease, asthma and cancer.

The consequences since 1992 have been 'a marked decline in surgical services; delays in diagnosis and treatment, a decline in the quality of hospital care and unnecessary suffering and premature death'.

That the system should survive is due to the firmly held socialist principles of the Castro government. Medical services are not com-

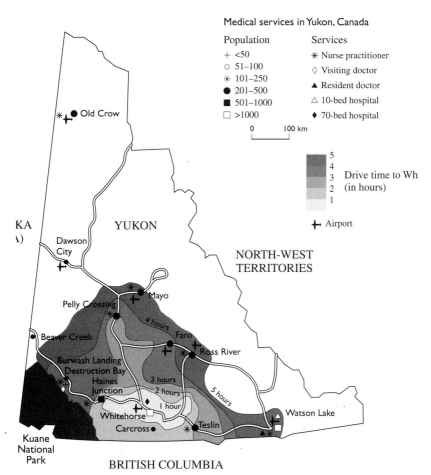

Figure 5.11 **Medical services in Yukon Canada**
(Source: Data from Yukon websites
http://199.247.156.23/cn/communities.htm)

mercial but are 'considered as one of the rights of humankind in modern society and should be freely accessible to everybody whatever their social economic and geographical position' (Radio Havana 2000).

Ways of maintaining an effective service are firstly to encourage a good diet: 'growing food is a much more pressing health problem than the ability to do heart transplants.'

There are 21 medical schools providing free training. All students must undertake three years 'social service medicine' in remote areas. Many doctors are 'exported' to other LEDCs. Complementary medicine includes the use of acupuncture to try to replace antibiotics, and herbal medicine. There is a strict moral regime and the incidence of

HIV/AIDS is low. Research institutes are concentrating their efforts on developing medicines from sugar cane products.

China

Can a proven system survive with the growth of capitalism?
Before the Communist Revolution of 1949, China was known for its high **infant mortality rate**. Malaria, typhoid, tuberculosis and other infectious diseases were widespread and the population:doctor ratio was over 7,000:1 (Meade and Earikson 2000).

In the new People's Republic, a massive health campaign was launched which was highly successful:

integrating traditional and Western medicine, simple paramedical training was given to peasants and soldiers. Instead of sending out teams of public health experts to halt disease and destroy pests, the entire populations of many areas were educated in such basic ideas as composting human waste to destroy pathogens or elimination of snails that transmit schistosomiasis.

The years of the Cultural Revolution from 1966–9 were very hard for those who were thought to oppose the government's ideas. Consequently, many professionals found themselves forced to work on labouring projects in remote rural areas, but the rural health programme, which began at that time, was revolutionary in a positive sense:

*   It was a three-tier system.
*   Primary healthcare was provided at village clinics through the **Barefoot Doctor** programme. Previously, any medical facilities might have been up to three days' walk away. The barefoot doctor was a local villager who had been given a brief training in order to attend to the community's needs, treating minor illnesses and promoting health and hygiene. Medicine was thus combined with farm work. Besides a doctor there were other health workers including midwives. About 2,000 people were served and the scheme was financed co-operatively.
*   In towns each clinic had around 16 healthcare workers and served between 15,000 to 50,000 people. Preventive medicine was also important here.
*   The top level was the county hospital, giving care to between 400,000 and 1.3 million people. This also supervised the town clinics.

By the late 1970s, 90% of all villages had such schemes. They were so successful that they became the model for community primary care in many other countries. Life expectancy rose to 71 years and IMR fell to 30/1,000 live births (1999). The more prosperous regions showed the greatest improvement.

Healthcare in China is now provided not only by the national system clinics but also has military and industrial sectors in addition to those for workers in other state services such as education. There has also been a rapid increase in wealth in rural areas and a demand for higher quality medical care. Many Barefoot Doctors could earn more by concentrating on farm work alone. Many doctors going from the state system into private practice have met this demand. This has led to 60% of rural health centres demanding fees. Only 5% of the rural population is still covered by the old system. Country dwellers often migrate to towns, as there they believe they can claim access to a range of superior services by right. Conversely, state sector employees are still very well served, as are the growing numbers of the new capitalist elite. Private healthcare is being encouraged, as is private medical insurance.

CIS

Has the fall of the former Soviet Union's rigid central planning made health-care more effective?
Before the Confederation of Independent States was created with the fall of communism in the early 1990s, the health service in the former Soviet Union was **centrally planned**. Health facilities were strictly allocated according to local government boundaries and population levels; there was no choice. The aim was to create a productive workforce. There were seven levels of care (Meade and Earikson 2000):

1. The central Ministry of Health, at the top, was responsible for 250 million people.
2. Republic ministries administered the areas of 5 million to 50 million people.
3. Regional health departments served 1 million to 5 million people.
4. The polyclinic served 40,000 to 150,000 people.
5. Urban neighbourhood clinics served up to 65,000 people.
6. Village clinics.
7. Clinics for farms

This vast system tried to provide a comprehensive service, with free treatment for half the population and the others paying merely for drugs and equipment. There were adequate numbers of health workers, but:

- the system was rigid and did not respond to local needs;
- those in high status jobs got much better treatment;
- the really privileged side-stepped the system to obtain maximum benefits;
- nearly all doctors were specialist, so primary care suffered badly: 'they (the doctors) do little more than treat viral illnesses, issue medical certificates and refer about half the cases they see to specialist colleagues.' Toon 1998;
- doctors were abundant but had a very low status and pay with consequent low morale: 'in Russia a doctor's pay is lower than the average wage and they earn more "moonlighting" as taxi drivers ' (Toon 1998);

- the more remote areas were given good facilities but despite incentives few doctors would go out to staff them;
- the whole system was dominated by an emphasis on keeping inputs high (such as numbers of health workers and hospital beds), rather than the quality of the care received and its effectiveness.

Despite this there were improvements in health; the IMR went down from 250/1,000 in 1900 to 20/1,000 in 1960.

Reforms to the system began in 1991 and aimed to de-centralise, with each regional government having more responsibility for decision-making. The funding was to be provided by compulsory social and state medical insurance (WHO 1999). Primary care and out-patient care was to be emphasised. In 1997, however, the income from the state insurance scheme funded only 35% of health expenditure. Arrears of contributions amounted to double the funding! This made the situation difficult as funding from regional authorities was drying up as soon as the insurance scheme began (from 100% in 1991 to 65% in 1997) (Shishkin 1998).

The basic health and welfare indicators reveal the detrimental effects on the population's health. The **death rate** went up from 11.3/1,000 in 1985 to 14.3/1,000 in 1996. **Life expectancy** fell from 69.3 to 65.9 over the same period. The reforms have a long way to go: 'Wide and sustained contact with democratic institutions and attitudes is needed if freedom is to grow and flourish in Russia' (Toon 1998).

2 Changing societies and future healthcare

a) Ageing population challenges

What is the problem?

In 1997, the WHO launched the Global Movement for Healthy Ageing:

> By 2020, the world will have more than 1 billion people age 60 and over and 710 million of them will live in developing countries ….The proportion of older people in the world's population will also continue to rise. Europe will retain the distinction of being the 'oldest' region, with the proportion of people 60 and over rising to 24% in 2020 form 19% today …. The 'oldest' country will be Japan with 31% of its population age 60 and over.

> People who reach old age in good health will be capable of contributing to society intellectually, spiritually and physically far beyond the age of 60. This is especially important given the projected demographic changes which would otherwise see a burgeoning number of people over 60 being regarded as a burden on health systems at a time of shrinking public health budgets.

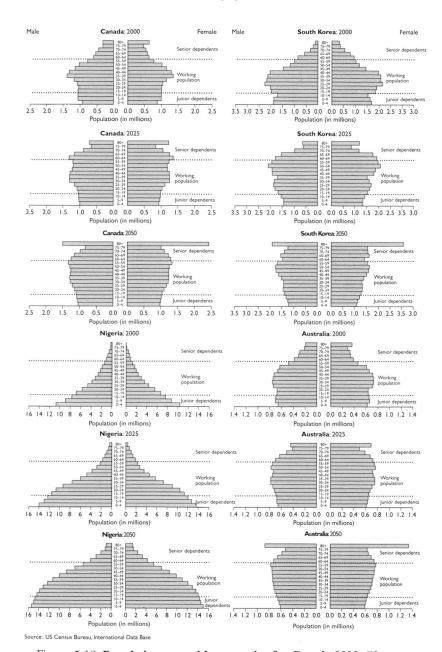

Source: US Census Bureau, International Data Base

Figure 5.12 **Population pyramid summaries for Canada 2000–50 an MEDC**
Population pyramid summaries for South Korea 2000–50 an NIC
Population pyramid summaries for Nigeria 2000–50 an LEDC
Population pyramid summary for Australia 2000–50 an MEDC

The following **social trends** make it even more important to plan carefully for an **ageing population** as traditional role of the female carer will be reduced by: more nuclear (parents and children only), rather than extended (grandparents, aunts, cousins) families; urbanisation; a higher proportion of women in the workforce; lack of social security schemes.

The **population pyramids** (Figure 5.12) graphically illustrate the shift in dependency ratios. The **senior dependency ratio** (the ratio of the number of people aged 65 and over to the number of working adults) is enlarged while the **junior dependency ratio** (the ratio of under 15 year olds to working adults) is falling (Rigg 1999).

How is it happening in MEDCs?
This process of ageing in MEDCs was influenced by the following factors (WHO 1998):

* in MEDCs ageing was gradual, as a result of a declining fertility rate and improving standards of living for most people after mass industrialisation;
* a much later development was the progress made in new and effective drugs and vaccines.

How is it happening in LEDCs?
In LEDCs the picture is different:

* population ageing is occurring due to rapid fertility decline;
* life expectancy was increased because of medical interventions using drugs and advanced technology;
* infectious diseases (as predicted by the epidemiological transition) have declined as a result of many interventions such as mass vaccination programmes and ORT;
* population ageing is often associated with poverty owing to inadequate family or welfare support;
* although traditional views of older people are that they are wise, these are in danger of being eroded by external influences.

The prospect of so many more people at risk from the **degenerative non-communicable diseases**, such as those of the circulatory system, cancers and diabetes, is a challenge to healthcare and welfare systems worldwide.

* In Cuba, 35% of men suffer from high blood pressure; cancer is responsible for around 30% of deaths in Latin America as a whole.
* Late onset diabetes affects 143 million people in the world.
* Mental health, especially forms of dementia, such as Alzheimer's disease, and depression will also be a problem. WHO estimates that there might be as many as 55 million people afflicted by senile dementia in LEDCs by 2020.
* Vision loss such as that caused by cataracts accounts for 40% of all blindness in LEDCs. While 1.35 million cataract operations are carried out in

the USA each year, the sophisticated technology needed is not available in the developing world. Thus, otherwise healthy people are made dependent.

The burden on LEDCs is worsened because they also have to contend with high rates of infectious diseases.

What is being done?

The WHO's programme on ageing and health addresses such issues as:

* establishing an adequate database about ageing for key decision-makers
* providing information to stimulate an awareness of the problem
* organising community-based programmes
* research, training and development.

The question of whether or not the growing number of elderly people will put an unbearable strain on the world economy is important (WHO 1999):

> There has been growing concern in many, particularly industrialised, countries about the levels of state expenditure for social protection ...This worldwide debate has unfortunately placed the entire emphasis on the cost to society of providing pensions and healthcare rather than on the continuing and significant economic contributions that older citizens make to society.

Two considerations are highlighted:

1. **Employment**: Most older people work after the age of 60 or 65, especially in those economies dominated by agriculture, until they are physically incapable of doing so. In Malawi 85% of men over 65 are still part of the workforce; in Liberia it is 70%. Old women who outlive their husbands in LEDCs are often forced to migrate to cities and become street hawkers as part of the informal economy (van der Gaag 1995). There is no biological reason for retirement at 60 or 65. Early withdrawal from the employment by older workers does not always mean job opportunities for those younger. Often older workers give stability and skill to the workforce. In Africa, especially where HIV/AIDS has produced so many orphans, grandmothers look after the children left behind.

2. **Pensions**: Many older people in MEDCs are covered by pensions from the public and private sectors to protect them from poverty. In an urbanised society with a mobile population this is essential, as informal care is scarce. If there were not state pension schemes more than 50% of the older MEDC population would be in poverty. This provision needs to be flexible, however, as resources will become increasingly limited. LEDCs do not often have this option. According to the World Bank, 60% of the world's workforce and 70% of old people are in the informal economy and without pension plans and unable to save.

In LEDCs, the inability to work through ill health or incapacity makes people unable to cover their subsistence requirements. In MEDCs, the unemployment associated with ill health creates insecurity. The WHO strongly advises a lifelong approach to healthcare to prevent such problems where possible.

Kasturi Sen, a specialist concerned with policies for ageing, suggests that a 'life-cycle' approach of preparing for old age by obtaining credit and buying land, especially for women, is vital. Better nutrition and contraception would improve later health.

> The growing number of older people who expect healthcare and old-age pensions should not be viewed as a threat or a crisis. ...It is the need to examine and make appropriate changes to health, social and economic policies, not the ageing of populations, that is the biggest challenge facing societies today.
>
> *WHO*, 1999

Ageing in MEDCs: estimating the distribution of the elderly and the demand for care

Canada

Of the total population, 3.7 million people, or 12.5% of the population is over 65. Of these, 380,000 are over 85, of whom 70.5% are female (Rosenberg 1998). The younger sector of this population is very different in its needs from the older. Most older Canadians live in the high-amenity areas in British Columbia and Ontario and in the newer suburbs of Toronto. Those wealthy and healthy enough to do so are able to move around in these zones. The demand for services is determined by their marital status and gender, in addition to their age. The institutions are mainly looking after those women over 85 who have lived alone and are in poor health. Rosenberg comments that 2031 will be the year of peak demand for homes, according to demographic projections.

Australia

The South Australian Network for Research on Ageing (SANRA) carried out extensive research on the distribution of older people in the state of South Australia in the late 1990s. This was particularly useful because a clearer picture can help in devising the appropriate level of care in order to keep old people in their homes for as long as possible, rather than using institutional care.

While South Australia's population has grown far more slowly than states such as Queensland and Western Australia, the proportion of those over 65 in the state has grown at a more rapid rate (from 8.5% in 1971 to 13.9% in 1996). Most of this growth has been in the ﾍlaide area. On retirement, people tend to move out of the city to ﾍe seaside settlements like Victor Harbour and Goolwa.

Specialist housing has made these towns even more popular with retired people; the rural areas have lost their older population as well as the city (only 1.8% of people over 65 live in rural areas). Within Australian cities as a whole there are some clear trends emerging in the distribution of older people:

* The central and inner suburbs seem to have high concentrations of older people, both in their own homes and in institutions.
* Seaside suburbs, although long-established, now attract older people due to purpose-built developments.
* The middle suburbs contain those immigrants from Europe in the 1950s and 1960s who stayed in close-knit communities in the area and are now of retirement age.
* The outer suburbs have a rapidly growing population but a smaller proportion is older.

The main characteristics of those parts of Adelaide with around 20% of the population over 65 are low-density suburbs with nucleated shopping centres, low public transport networks and few services for the elderly. There is a marked outward shift in the pattern in the city generally. There are concentrations of people over 75 in the middle suburbs where it is easy to plan efficient Meals on Wheels services, for instance.

In non-metropolitan resort areas in Australia as a whole, older people are to be found living in settlements along the southern and northern coast of New South Wales due to the attractive scenery and equable climate. Country towns tend to attract retired farm workers who use the improved facilities but maintain their former social networks more easily than they would in a larger town.

Population forecasts for the proportion of elderly people in Australia (see Figure 5.12d) suggest the median age of the population will rise from 34 to 46 in 2051.The figures for South Australia are 40 to 51 in 2051. The proportion of those over 65 will rise from 14% to 31% in 2051. Those aged 75 and over will be 16.5% of the population by 2051.

All these trends 'must not be seen as problems. They present opportunities and challenges and these must be identified and taken up.'

USA

America's elderly population is now growing at a moderate pace. But not too far into the future, the growth will become rapid. So rapid, in fact, that by the middle of the next century, it might be completely inaccurate to think of ourselves as a Nation of the Young; there could be more persons who are elderly (65 or over) than young (14 or younger).

Frank Hobbs, *Sixty-five plus in the United States*, US Department of Commerce, May 1995

In 1900, one in 25 of the US population was over 65. In 1994 it was one in eight. In 2020 the elderly population will more than double, mainly because those born after the Second World War ('baby boomers') will be entering old age. The 'oldest old', those over 85, were 10% of the elderly population in 1994. Life expectancy has risen from 35 in 1900 to 76 in 1994. The racial mix in the US means that 36% of the elderly will be black or Hispanic.

Women tend to live longer than men. The ratio of males to females is 3:2 at age 65 but is 5:2 by the age of 85. Elderly men also tend to be married, whereas elderly women are more likely to be living alone. This means that the women are more vulnerable when frail and unwell. A survey in 1992 revealed that 75% of those over 65 and 66% of those over 75 considered themselves to be in good health.

Nonetheless, there are many elderly people who need help with daily tasks as they suffer from illnesses and chronic conditions such as arthritis. Half of those over 85 needed help in 1990. This means that there are going to be more and more relatives, usually female and in their 50s and 60s, who will have to care for them. The ratio of very elderly (over 85) to middle-aged potential carers will go up from 10:100 in 1993 to 29:100 in 2050.

Seven out of ten of those who died in 1991 in the US were over 65. Most of theses deaths were from heart disease, cancer or stroke.

Poverty is a problem for elderly people but there is great variation between racial groups and between the sexes (see Figure 5.13). Female blacks appear to be at most risk; white men were least affected. The better educated also survive longer and with a higher income, which is not surprising. The educational background of the elderly will be better in years to come as high-school graduates will

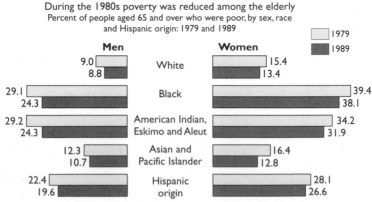

Figure 5.13 **During the 1980s, poverty was reduced among the elderly**
(Source: ibid)

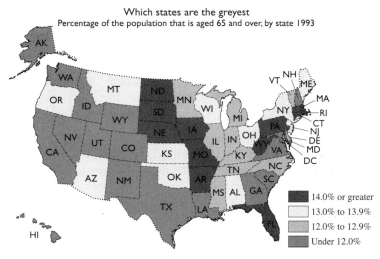

Figure 5.14 **Which states are the greyest?**
(Source: Ibid.)

form a larger proportion of them. Only 12% of the elderly had college degrees in 1993 whereas 27% of those in their 40s had them.

As one of the states with the highest populations, California had the greatest *number* of elderly people in 1994, with 3 million. Florida is also densely populated and has the greatest *percentage* of old people (19%). Many people migrate to Florida on retirement and thus the concentration of services for the elderly will have to increase. However, those in urban poverty who cannot afford to move to the 'sunshine states' will be in greater need of support (Figure 5.14).

Ageing in NICs: the benefits of pension planning

Those Asian NICs with **mature population structures** (see Figure 5.12b) such as Hong Kong, Singapore, South Korea and Taiwan will experience **rapid demographic ageing** by 2010 (Rigg 1999). Later, by 2050, China, Indonesia and Thailand, for instance, will have the same experience.

Since the young no longer feel the obligation to look after elderly relatives as was always the case with previous generations, support for the increasingly large numbers of old people will be difficult. Old people living with their families (**co-residence**) now make up over half the elderly population in Asia; this will decline. The valuable work done by grandparents in the home will thereby be lost.

Pension schemes are more common in the 'mature' NICs such as South Korea, where most of the population is covered. This is much less in China (40%) and Thailand (10%), for example. But those 'fully-funded' schemes which earmark an individual's contributions for their retirement, as in Singapore, will put far less strain on a country's economy than the 'pay-as-you-go' systems in South Korea where current contributions have to fund benefits.

Other sources of care such as non-governmental organisations (NGOs) include Cambodia's HelpAge and Singapore's Tsao Foundation. The Singapore government has also passed the Maintenance of Parents Bill in 1994 giving rights to parents over 60 to demand maintenance from their children.

Treating the increased incidence of degenerative diseases, which are more expensive to treat than fighting infections, is also a challenge.

The high proportion of economically active people was one of the factors which assisted the rapid economic growth in Asia. This trend will change as **dependency ratios** shift and the **senior dependency ratio** increases. Rigg comments:

> It is important to put in place policies to anticipate demo-
> graphic ageing, and to realise the economic and human poten-
> tial of this growing segment of the population. These measures
> are needed to avoid a situation where the elderly are margin-
> alised at the edges of society and economy.

Ageing in an LEDC: Nigeria: what happens when the extended family breaks down?

Elizabeth Obadina (1995) describes the situation thus:

> daughters were bullied into caring for elderly parents, aunts,
> uncles or even cousins by well-organised associations of elderly
> people in the village. Nowadays, a sense of duty is not one of the
> values encouraged by Nigerian society, the youth aren't to hand
> in the villages and our elders are losing out.

Most Nigerians, unless they are lucky to have saved and bought some land, have to work to support themselves. If and when their health fails, they are reduced to living on the streets. Lagos has a population of over 6 million but only two old peoples' homes for 37 destitute old people. Nigeria has 13 homes in all for a population of over 95 million.

The Holy Family home for the elderly in Lagos makes exhaustive attempts to re-unite elderly people with their families, but it is not always successful as those families are themselves struggling. Ideally, old people would like to live in their ancestral village; many who can afford it build houses room by room while they are still living in the city. This is because they fear urban social isolation.

However, many older couples are split; the husband working to support his possibly grown-up family and living in rented rooms in a town while his wife, who may well be frail, looks after the house in the village back home. What money she has is sent as a remittance from her husband; farming covers her food requirements only. 'Pensionless, confronted with increasingly expensive healthcare and with family resources stretched to the limit, all Nigerians face a grim old age unless the Government steps in with material help.'

There are moves to persuade the Government to provide free healthcare for those over 65. In northern Nigeria, households are being subsidised to keep their destitute elderly relatives from begging on the streets.

The younger population is reluctant to contribute to pensions. Older people have a low priority at the moment as life expectancy until the late 1980s was around 60 years. Immunisation for children is still seen as a more important social need.

> so, care for the elderly is where it has always been – in the bosom of the family...to Nigeria's cash-strapped government this makes both financial and ideological sense. The problem is that the elderly are getting a raw deal from the very bosom that is meant to sustain them.
>
> Elizabeth Obadina, 1995

What of the future?

There are reports from the University of Chicago which suggest that the progressive lengthening of life expectancy cannot continue indefinitely (Henderson 2001). People in countries such as France, the UK and the USA may well have a life expectancy of 100 in the twenty-second century. In some more advanced LEDCs, people may live to 85. Jay Olshansky comments, however;

> Future gains in life expectancy will eventually be measured in days or months rather than in years...it is sobering to realise that life expectancy could actually decline for some populations because of the re-emergence of infectious diseases, social and political unrest, or natural disasters.

b) Welfare issues: the homelessness crisis

This study of homelessness in the UK is but one aspect of the range of important welfare issues confronting MEDCs. The effects of home-lessness in the UK and in LEDCs have been discussed in the sections on refugees in Chapter 2, poverty and access to care in Chapter 3 and in care for the elderly earlier in this chapter.

What action has been taken?

The UK government introduced the Rough Sleepers Initiative (RSI) in the late 1990s. It is: 'a multi-agency effort to provide temporary and permanent accommodation to people sleeping rough in central London.' (UNESCO report)

The scheme targeted five areas where **rough sleeping** was a particular problem in London, for example the Strand. It was also linked to a government initiative for spreading good practice in helping the homeless in other areas in the UK (the RSU – Rough Sleepers Unit).

As part of the White Paper outlining the health strategy 'Our Healthier Nation' in 1999, the government also produced an expert report from the Health Development Agency (HDA) which considered the opportunities and barriers for promoting the health of the homeless (HDA 2000). The following factors were identified:

1. To be homeless means being isolated without accommodation, being vulnerable and unemployed.
2. The homeless are well aware of the negative impact of their situation on the state of their health and yet find it hard to remedy.
3. Improving the health and well-being of the homeless can range from providing simply food and shelter to tackling the determinants of homelessness such as housing policy, social exclusion and provision for those leaving care.
4. Healthcare services are difficult for the homeless to access and should therefore be more flexible in their approach and cover all types of homelessness.
5. There should be far more collaboration between agencies involved in health promotion.
6. Any programmes to help the homeless should be carefully evaluated.

Outcry (Summer 2000), the newsletter for health action for the homeless, describes the introduction of Personal Medical Service pilot schemes, which give GPs a flexible way of responding to local health needs. These are now in place to help the homeless in Lambeth, Southwark and Lewisham. The RSU specified that GPs must offer the homeless equal access to primary health care but delivery has obviously been a problem. Lester (2000) points out that 36% of homeless people in a recent survey had difficulty registering with a GP and 84% preferred a specialist homeless medical service, but suggests that this might be because they had experienced refusal from conventional practices.

Hopkinson House, a project in Vauxhall, South London, to provide accommodation, support and resettlement for homeless drinkers, drug users and people with mental illness has successfully used a multi-agency approach. The project costs £1 million a year, funded by Westminster City Council; and Kensington, Chelsea and Westminster health authorities and has helped people to 'de-tox' and even to move into their own flats.

Health risks

One of the most serious aspects of homelessness is the likelihood of contracting tuberculosis (TB). This is compounded by the use of drugs and, of course, HIV/AIDS infection. There is some concern that TB will be much more prominent in London if the health of the homeless is not carefully monitored. Certainly, the possibility of successful DOTS treatment is much reduced if the patient has no fixed abode.

c) Combating new and emergent diseases

Chapter 4 discusses the rise of new and resistant strains of infectious disease, which will put an undoubted strain on the global healthcare system. A WHO report (November 2000) points out the main problems:

1. Globalisation of infectious diseases is more and more of a problem due to: increased migration; increased tourism; growth in the trade of food products; social and environmental changes linked to urbanisation, deforestation and climate change; changes in food processing methods, such as those which produced BSE.
2. Intentional or deliberate release of infectious agents, for example anthrax spores.
3. The need for international co-operation to prevent mis-information, over-reaction to media coverage and insufficient capacity at national level to recognise diseases and to contain them effectively.

The WHO has maintained these objectives since it was founded in 1948, and is now strengthened by the International Health Regulations.

Some recent examples of the need to be vigilant include:

- The importing of yellow fever, which is fatal, into the USA and Switzerland in 1996 by tourists who had not had yellow fever vaccinations returning from areas where the disease was endemic.
- The occurrence of 10,000 cases of malaria imported into the EU in· 1996, 25% of which were in the UK.
- The re-emergence of the El Tor cholera strain in Peru in 1991, which led to 3,000 deaths, the cessation of sea-food exports and the loss of tourist revenue.

In MEDCs the main concern is to prevent the diseases from entering but in LEDCs the aim is to detect outbreaks early in order to stop their mortality, spread and negative effects on tourism. An effective **surveillance system** is of paramount importance. This was set up in 1996 linking networks of laboratories and medical centres in all 191 counties belonging to the WHO. There is now a weekly epidemiological record of infectious diseases.

The trends which will influence the effectiveness of control measures, according to Cliff, Haggett and Smallman-Raynor (1998) include:

- the lack of physical barriers now that air travel is now universal
- the ability to transmit details of reported incidence rapidly via the Internet
- the replacement of total reporting with sampling owing to the increasing number of disease outbreaks to be monitored

- the use of mathematical modelling to highlight anomalies (unusual patterns) in automatic recording systems
- the relationship between disease control and socio-economic development: 'the world's most ruthless killer and the greatest cause of suffering on earth …is extreme poverty.'

d) The role of international organisations

WHO

One of the most prominent organisations promoting health worldwide is the World Health Organisation (WHO), based in Geneva, which is a specialised section of the United Nations (UN). In addition to reporting on health from its regional offices which cover its 191 member states, it also produces an annual report on a specific theme which is backed up by exhaustive statistical appendices. The themes for the last few years:

2000 – health systems (see Chapter 3)
1999 – providing modern health care for all
1998 – global targets for health in 2000
1997 – the problem of ageing

Other activities include its global vaccination programmes discussed in Chapter 4 and its fact sheets on all aspects of health and disease. Without its co-ordinating role in monitoring disease globally there would have been little progress in infectious disease elimination; in addition, future challenges will be impossible to meet without its involvement. Its enormous website is mentioned in the references section.

UNICEF

UNICEF, the United Nations Children's Fund, was founded at the end of the Second World War 'to relieve the suffering of children in war-torn Europe'. Since then it has responded to many crises affecting children's health, such as helping to eradicate polio and supporting children with HIV/AIDS. It funds programmes:

- to help prevent childhood illnesses and death
- to encourage care and stimulation for young children
- to make pregnancy and childbirth safe
- to help with girls' education and female equality.

In its 2000 report, Kofi Annan, secretary-general of the UN, commented on UNICEF's work in upholding the convention on the Rights of the Child, which came into existence in 1989. Other work mentioned in the report is UNICEF's part in co-ordinating the polio vaccine programme (for 9 million children in the Democratic Republic of the Congo alone). HIV/AIDS and its current and future effects on sub-Saharan Africa in particular continues to be a major challenge. Helping children survive the first few years of life involves providing clean water, monitoring growth, advising on adequate nutrition, immunisation, ORT, and the treatment of acute respiratory infections. Health workers in many parts of the world are given extra training in these fields.

Dealing with more than 13 million children who had been orphaned by HIV/AIDS by the end of 1999 was a key priority. Around 1.3 million children had HIV/AIDs at the end of 1999, most of them in sub-Saharan Africa. UNICEF works to support them directly and in education programmes, especially for girls, as an important part of its prevention strategy.

Summary

1. All healthcare was once privately funded. Now it is financed in many other ways, which include tax and social security systems, employers' contributions, charities and NGOs.
2. The poor often fail to obtain adequate care.
3. Governments have many different priorities when it comes to health spending.
4. Field's model of healthcare types classifies them according to the organisation of their resources, their financing and the degree of state participation.
5. Emergent healthcare is shown in LEDCs such as those in tropical Africa and India.
6. Pluralistic healthcare exists in the USA.
7. Insurance/social security care in France tops the WHO effectiveness league table.
8. National Health Services exist in the UK and in Canada.
9. Canada has different methods of organising its national health service in each province.
10. Socialised care in Cuba fits the communist ideal of healthcare for all.
11. China had a most effective socialised care organisation with its Barefoot Doctor scheme which revolutionised rural healthcare.
12. The CIS had a rigid system of socialised medicine before the former Soviet Union disappeared in 1990.
13. Ageing populations will be the greatest health challenge in the twenty-first century. By 2020 there will be more than 1 billion people aged 60 and over; 75% of these will be in LEDCs.
14. The epidemiological transition suggests that there will be a rise in degenerative diseases as a consequence. Since these are more difficult to treat effectively than infectious diseases this will put further strain on healthcare and welfare systems.
15. Older people can still be productive workers, but financial security from a pension is denied to 60% to 70% of the world's workforce.
16. In MEDCs such as Canada, Australia and the USA, there are areas where there is a high concentration of older people.

17. In NICs those with earmarked pension schemes will not fear financial insecurity in old age.
18. LEDCs, such as Nigeria, face the biggest problem.
19. Homelessness is an important welfare issue in MEDCs.
20. Another future health challenge is the growth of new and emergent diseases, such as BSE and TB.
21. International organisations such as the WHO and UNICEF have played a vital role in improving health worldwide since the 1950s.

Suggested essay title

How best can health and welfare be funded in the future?

The section at the end of Chapter 2 gives general advice for essay writing. It should be consulted in addition to these more specific hints.

Choice of title

- *'How best'* implies that there is a range of options, but that it is possible to identify one that could be best.
- The models here are Field's Model of health care types, the Epidemiological Transition and WHO's new universalism of primary care.

Research

- The chart for this chapter gives you the opportunity to choose contrasting types of healthcare system to investigate.
- The WHO Report 2000 is worth consulting for background information.
- Each case study needs background details about its particular future challenges.
- Be sure you have clear definitions of *health* and *welfare* as the whole essay depends on them!
- What are the main sources of funding in general and in your case study areas in particular?

Planning

- You will need to decide how effective each method of health care funding actually seems to be for the future. It might be a good idea to rank the ones you have chosen to study according to the criteria given by the WHO Report.
- Also consider the uses of the funding such as resources and provision.
- You should be numbering the links on your diagram (according to the ranking you have given health care systems) to help you to order the paragraphs in the essay or report.
- There is no one right answer here.
- Summary spider diagrams are probably the best way of showing funding contrasts.

References used and bibliography

Books

Advanced texts

If you get hold of any of these you will be in the 'serious student' category! They are all above the standard A2 level text. They will have to be obtained on special loan from your library.

Cliff, A. & Haggett, P. (1992) *Atlas of Disease Distributions*, Blackwell, Oxford
Cliff, A., Haggett, P. & Smallman-Raynor, M. (1998) *Deciphering Global Epidemics*, CUP, Cambridge
Burglary Prevention, *Crime Reduction Programme* Home Office, 1999
Elliot, P., Wakefield, J., Best, N. & Briggs, D. (2000) *Spatial Epidemiology*, OUP, Oxford
Meade, M. & Earickson, R. (2000) *Medical Geography*, The Guildford Press, New York
Pearce, D. & Crooks, C. (1999) *Twyford: Ringing the Changes*, George Mann, Winchester
Thubron, C. (2000) *In Siberia*, Penguin, London
Whitehead, M. (1992) *The Health Divide*, Penguin, London
Wilkinson, R. (1996) *Unhealthy Societies*, Routledge, London and New York
Wrench, G. (1924) *Chavasse's Advice to a Mother*, J. & A. Churchill, London

Texts accessible for A2

McCormick, J. & Fisher-Hoch, S. (1996) *The Virus Hunters*, Bloomsbury, London
Wills, C. (1996) *Plagues*, HarperCollins, London

Journals, Newspapers, Magazines and other documents (specific editions)

British Heart Foundation News, Spring 1997
British Medical Journal 308:1125–1128 1994, 314:591 1998, 317:714–4, 319:995–997, 320:563–566, 1687, 321:563–565, 726 391:1162–1165 1999
Chrysalis Journal, Johns Hopkins School of Medicine, 1999
Croatian Medical Journal 39, 3 September 1998
The Economist, 24 February 2001
Emerging Infectious Diseases vol. 4(3) 1998, vol. 6(1) February 2000
Epidemiology 11:1, 11:4 July 2000, 11:5, 12:1 January 2001
Financial Times, December 2000
The Geographical Magazine, July 1995
Geography Review, March 1999, January 2001
Independent, 29 November 2000
Independent, 25 November 1996

Journal of Epidemiology & Community Health, 54 404–408, 411–413, 745–749, 750–755, 890–898, 923–929
The Lancet, 342 1993, September 25 1999, 354 2047 1999
The New Internationalist, October (1995), 264 (1995), 280 (1996), 1998, 326 (August 2000)
New Statesman, 18 September 1998
New Zealand Herald, 1 November 2000
People and the Planet, 4 1995, 6: 3 1997, 7:1 1998
The Pharmaceutical Journal, 285 7183, 1 July 2000
PPP Healthcare leaflet PB16558a/10
Royal College of General Practitioners, discussion document 1998, January 2000
SANRA – the center for ageing studies, Flinders University of South Australia, 1998
Sociology Review, September 1993
Sunday Telegraph, 24 January 1999
The Times, 2 December 1996, 12 March 1997, 27 November 1997, 5 December 1997, 6 March 2000, 26 September 2000, 21 November 2000, 29 November 2000, 30 November 2000, 6 February 2001, 7 February 2001, 10 February 2001, 16 February 2001, 19 February 2001, 26 February 2001, 12 March 2001, 20 March 2001, 22 March 2001, 3 April 2001, 5 April 2001, 20 April 2001
US Dept of Commerce, 1995
The Week, 4 November 2000, 16 December 2000, 10 February 2001, 17 March 2001
WHO: Health in Europe 1997, Global Movement for Healthy Ageing 1997, *Highlights on Health in the Russian Federation 1999*, World Health Day 1999, *World Health Report 2000*, Global Health Security-Epidemic Alert and Response 2000
Winchester News Extra 47, 15 February 2001
World's Children, Save the Children 1997

Journals, Newspapers, Magazines and other documents (general)

Newspapers – the website for each paper also has search facilities (also available on CD-ROM):
The Times, Guardian, Independent, Daily Telegraph, Financial Times, Daily Mail

If not in your library, the following are all easily available either at newsagents or on the Internet: *The Week, Geographical Magazine, The Economist, New Scientist, New Internationalist, People and the Planet* (on the web), Area (RGs), Geo Factsheet, Geofile.

These may well be in your school or college library, they are also available from the publishers, Philip Allan: *Geographical Review, Sociology Review*. If you want some more serious medical details, try these. The *BMJ* is surprisingly easy to read. The *Journal of Epidemiology & Community Health* and *Epidemiology* have many papers on diseases in relation to environmental factors but are hard to obtain outside your local teaching hospital library, although they do have websites.

Websites

As sites frequently appear and disappear, it is best to list here those of large organizations, which should be fairly reliable long term. As a general search facility, **www.google.com** works very efficiently.

- **www.who.int** – the World Health Organisation site is so massive that you might find you never need anything else! It has **statistics** (/whosis), **tropical disease control** (/ctd), epidemic monitoring (/outbreak), **HIV/AIDS data** (emc-hiv/factsheets) and **environmental health** (/peh-emf) sections. Its annual reports are accompanied by a wealth of data. Its European branch in Copenhagen (.dn) has specific reports on different countries.
- **www.chi.com** – the US Centre for International Health information gives health information on many different countries.
- **www.census.gov/ipc** – this has an international data base (mainly socio-economic and population). You can have a wonderful time creating age/sex population pyramids for any country in the world and projecting them into the future as far as 2050 (/ipc/www/idbpyr.html). The dependency ratios are worrying.
- **www.cdc.gov** – this is the US Centres for Disease Control and Prevention site. It has information on emerging diseases (/EID), infectious diseases (/ncid) and other health data for the US.
- **www.statistics.gov.uk** – this has information on the UK 2001 census.
- **www.nhs.uk/nationalplan/summary** – this gives background on the UK NHS plan from July 2000.
- **www.odci.gov/cia/publications/factbook** – if you want to know anything about any country in the world, turn to this – the World Factbook.
- **www.worldbank.org** – studies of Health Nutrition and Poverty undertaken by the World Bank in 54 LEDCs (/hnp) and on Equity, Poverty and Health (/poverty/health/data/guide). Mainly databases.
- **www.ciesin.org** – this is the Center for International Earth Science Information Network, which has detailed information about climatic change and its effects on health.
- **www.bbc.co.uk** – BBC news on-line has a wealth of health-related news stories, a good archive search facility and a very useful list of links with other related sites for whatever topic you are interested in.
- **www.geog.queensu.ca/Rosenberg/** – Mark Rosenberg is a Canadian medical geographer and this is his course, mainly as a series of slide shows. It gives some very useful background and case studies, but remember that it is for University students!
- **www.geocities.com/Tokyo/Flats/7335/medical_geography.htm** – quite an eccentric address, but it is a most comprehensive introduction to the subject, clear and user-friendly.